Expect the Best

Expect the Best

Your Guide to Healthy Eating Before, During, and After Pregnancy

Elizabeth M. Ward, M.S., R.D.

WILEY

John Wiley & Sons, Inc.

Published by John Wiley & Sons, Inc., Hoboken, New Jersey

Published simultaneously in Canada

The information contained in this book is not intended to serve as a replacement for professional medical advice. Any use of the information in this book is at the reader's discretion. The author and the publisher specifically disclaim any and all liability arising directly or indirectly from the use or application of any information contained in this book. A health care professional should be consulted regarding your specific situation.

For general information about our other products and services, please contact our Customer Care Department within the United States at (800) 762-2974, outside the United States at (317) 572-3993 or fax (317) 572-4002.

Wiley also publishes its books in a variety of electronic formats. Some content that appears in print may not be available in electronic books. For more information about Wiley products, visit our web site at www.wiley.com.

ISBN 978-0-470-29076-7

Printed in the United States of America

10 9 8 7 6 5 4 3 2

Contents

Foreword

Everyone knows how important it is to have a healthy diet when you're eating for two. As a pediatrician and former director of a newborn nursery, I have fielded a variety of questions about healthy eating both during and right after pregnancy—is it safe to eat sushi, can I drink caffeine (or alcohol), and what do I do if I can't swallow those huge prenatal vitamins? Perhaps most importantly, many new parents just want to know how to give their child the best start in life. I'm thrilled that I can now refer my patients to *Expect the Best*, which covers all of the concerns mentioned above and a whole lot more.

Pregnancy is a time when many women change their eating and lifestyle habits for the better and often continue these healthy habits as their children grow. Since pregnancy isn't always planned, however, all of the sixty-three million women of childbearing age in the United States would do well to be as fit and healthy as possible, even before they become pregnant. Not only does a pregnant woman's nutrition affect her own weight, health, and chances for shedding those pregnancy pounds soon after birth, but it can also significantly affect her baby's health—both at the time of delivery and as her child grows into adulthood.

Consider the fact that the current generation of children is overfed yet undernourished, and is at risk for obesity, heart disease, diabetes, and high blood pressure as early as the preteen years. Because of their poor health habits, this generation is also the first in recent times that may not live as long as their parents. More than four million babies are born every year, and focusing on pregnancy nutrition and lifestyle can make a significant positive contribution to the health of these children.

In this new comprehensive resource by Elizabeth Ward and the American Dietetic Association, parents-to-be can find extensive, up-to-date information to help them make the best choices about nutrition, exercise, and food safety. *Expect the Best* discusses how many extra calories are really necessary when you're pregnant or breastfeeding a baby. And unlike many other books on pregnancy and nutrition, this one uniquely addresses the role a father's nutrition plays on the future health of a child.

You will learn about the relationships between diet and fetal development during pregnancy as well as complications such as fertility problems and premature births. In addition, you will understand the roles multivitamin supplements and exercise can play on preventing birth defects, excess weight gain, and other medical problems. Because many Americans do not get the recommended thirty minutes of physical activity daily, *Expect the Best* describes manageable ways to build exercise into one's usual routine.

Many families are opting for organic foods to avoid pesticides or are concerned about bacteria in raw or undercooked foods, contaminants in drinking water, as well as the mercury content of different types of fish. This guide discusses the numerous food safety considerations during the childbearing years, pregnancy, and while breast-feeding. In addition, there are millions of Americans who have adopted a vegetarian diet; this book teaches them how, during pregnancy, to get enough protein, iron, calcium, and other nutrients traditionally found in meat products.

Finally, sleep-deprived and time-starved parents are always looking for nutrient-rich and easy-to-prepare meal ideas. As a means to control portion size and ingredients, making one's own food at home can be key to maintaining a healthy weight, not to mention saving money. *Expect the*

Best offers useful nutrition information for more than fifty recipes that don't skimp on flavor or require hours in the kitchen—allowing you as an expectant or new parent more time to concentrate on caring for yourself and your baby.

—Jennifer Shu, M.D., pediatrician,
editor of *Baby and Child Health*, and
coauthor of *Heading Home with
Your Newborn* and *Food Fights*

Acknowledgments

All books are a group effort, this book even more so.

The information in *Expect the Best* is backed by the nearly seventy thousand members of the American Dietetic Association, the nation's largest group of nutrition professionals. Thirteen of those members, all registered dietitians with expertise in pregnancy nutrition, reviewed *Expect the Best*, pointing out how to improve the book to make it the most recent, most reliable, and most accurate resource about pregnancy and nursing on bookshelves. For their time and expertise, I am grateful to the following: Denise Andersen, M.S., R.D., L.D., C.L.C.; Heather Baden, M.S., R.D., C.D.N.; Mary D. Brown, M.S., R.D., L.D.N.; Miriam Erick, M.S., R.D., C.D.E., L.D.N.; Sumiti Gupta, R.D.; Gina Jarman Hill, Ph.D., R.D.,L.D.; Amy C. Huelle, R.D., C.D.E.; Melinda Johnson, M.S., R.D.; Maggie McHugh, M.S., R.D., C.D.N.; Julie M. Moreschi, M.S., R.D., L.D.N.; Gita Patel, M.S., R.D., C.D.E., L.D.; Judy D. Simon, M.S., R.D., C.D., C.H.E.S.; and Joanne Volpe, M.S., R.D.

In addition, I am thankful for the mothers who talked with me about their pregnancy experiences. Their insightful, and often humorous, remarks, scattered throughout *Expect the Best*, will help women to better follow the advice offered in this book and help them to get through any rough patches during pregnancy and when nursing.

I would also like to thank the American Dietetic Association's Laura Pelehach, an editor who offered the good sense and the patience that's required for turning any manuscript into a book. And, speaking of patience, thanks, as always, to my husband and three daughters, who saw me through yet another book-writing adventure. Thanks, too, to my mother, Anne, who offered her support and recipe-testing expertise.

Introduction

This is your first pregnancy, and having a baby is new to you. Perhaps you're an experienced parent, but you haven't had a child in years, and you're wondering what's new. You could be nursing an infant and thinking of having another baby sometime soon. Whatever the situation, this book is for every woman (and her male partner) in her childbearing years.

Just the fact that you picked up this book means that you are taking an important first step: doing what you can now to help your unborn child on the road to a healthy future. An increasing body of evidence shows that eating the right foods, starting well before you even conceive, can have an enormous affect on the future health of your child.

As a future or new mother, you want to do the right thing. I know; I've been there. Not only am I a registered dietitian, I am the mother of three. I remember well those anxious early days, wondering what I could do to ensure that my children would be healthy and happy. As a working woman and a mother, I found that it was not always easy or possible to abide by expert advice while juggling my career, family, and social life. With this in mind, when I began writing this book, I made it my goal to blend the most recent scientific research about having a baby and nursing a child with practical insights and easy-to-adhere-to tips and advice. I wanted to create a one-stop guide that would show expectant mothers how to nurture themselves and their unborn children and one that they could refer to again and again.

In *Expect the Best*, you'll find the most up-to-date advice about how and what to eat during this exciting time in your life. I will walk you through a healthy lifestyle from before pregnancy to the months after delivery, and I will help you to answer the questions "What should I be eating?" and "How much physical activity do I need?" no matter what stage of life you're in. You can be assured that in this book you'll find the latest scientific information you can trust. All of the information between these covers is backed up by the nearly seventy thousand members of the American Dietetic Association.

Experts make exciting inroads every day into understanding how you—and your partner—can have the healthiest baby possible. For example, more than ever is known about the role that fathers play in their future babies' health. Men who think that their contribution to making a baby begins and ends at conception should think again; experts now say that a man's health habits prior to his partner's pregnancy influence his child's well-being more than was previously believed. Did you know that research suggests that a man's body weight influences his chances of fathering a child? So does his consumption of folic acid, a B vitamin that women are encouraged to take in their childbearing years to prevent birth defects. Having a child is more of a partnership than you may have thought.

In addition, medical advances have made it possible for many couples to work through their fertility problems and conceive a child when they were not able to in the past. In fact, according to recent scientific evidence, when a woman eats a balanced diet and follows other healthy habits, she increases her chances of pregnancy through assisted reproduction, such as in vitro fertilization. More than ever, women are delivering healthy babies well into their forties; eating right and engaging in regular physical activity make an older woman's pregnancy smoother by helping her to avoid such complications as diabetes and high blood pressure. In fact, a balanced diet and the right amount of exercise can help mothers of all ages—whether they are carrying one child, twins, triplets, or more—with these issues and with other chronic conditions that can complicate pregnancies.

Getting Primed for Pregnancy

Years ago, women waited for a positive pregnancy test to quit smoking, stop drinking, and eat better. That attitude is old hat. Ideally, you should work with your doctor, nurse practitioner, or certified nurse-midwife and registered dietitian to adopt positive habits and get a handle on chronic conditions well before conception in order to head off the complications that could decrease fertility and jeopardize pregnancy.

The sooner you start working on your health, the better. More than half of the pregnancies in the United States are unexpected, so you need to be prepared for pregnancy when you least expect it. Once you're pregnant, you become your child's sole source of nourishment. You don't have an endless reserve of nutrients that a baby can draw from to grow and develop; every day you need to replenish your reserve with foods that give you the most nutrition for the calories. But no worries; it's not as overwhelming as it sounds. A healthy diet prior to pregnancy ensures that you have the nutrients "on board" once pregnancy starts, which is why *Expect the Best*, like no other pregnancy book on the shelves today, emphasizes getting in shape before conceiving a child. If your diet wasn't so great before you got pregnant, don't sweat it. Just take it from here, eating what you need for the stage you're in now.

The Power of Diet

Imagine that you could head off heart disease, diabetes, high blood pressure, obesity, and other persistent problems in your child, armed with a single weapon: your fork. This might sound impossible, but it's not.

The notion that a mother can "program" her child's health with what she eats may seem far-fetched, but it's gaining ground. Understanding how the environment in the womb influences lifelong well-being is an exciting area of medical research that keeps turning up new discoveries.

Here's an example of the power of food choices. When pregnant women fail to eat enough, are lacking in certain nutrients, or both, they set the stage for chronic conditions in their son or daughter years down the road. The theory is that an undernourished developing baby diverts sparse energy and nutrients to areas that really need it at the time, like the brain, at the expense of other vital organs, like the kidneys and the heart. Spreading nutrients thin permanently alters a person's metabolism and organ function, and this can increase the risk of such conditions as high blood pressure and heart disease years later in your child.

Preterm Birth: A Pressing Problem

Although researchers are poised to find out even more about the subtle relationships between diet and fetal development, problems remain. Preterm birth is particularly persistent.

Preterm birth occurs when a woman delivers a child before the thirty-seventh week of pregnancy. Every year, more than five hundred thousand babies are born in the United States before their time. Perhaps you've delivered a child before your due date; in that case, you know why being born early is problematic. Preterm infants are prone to complications at birth (and beyond) that often require specialized attention for months or years. It's not possible to prevent every preterm birth, of course. However, healthy living is one of the best strategies for taking your pregnancy to term.

Your Guide to a Healthy Pregnancy

Even if you're already eating well and engaging in regular physical activity, this book has plenty else to offer. Almost everything you need to know about what to do before, during, and after pregnancy is included in these pages, and it's not limited to food and nutrition. *Expect the Best* includes the latest information from the country's top health organizations about how much to exercise, what vaccinations you need before conception, why you should quit smoking, how lifestyle affects a couple's chances for conception, and even how your dental health influences your pregnancy. As an added bonus, the book includes tips and stories about everything from morning sickness to losing the pregnancy pounds from women who have been there. Here's a preview of what's in the pages ahead:

- Why you need to have a thorough medical examination prior to pregnancy and the blood tests you should request from your doctor
- The importance of achieving and maintaining a healthy weight before pregnancy, how much weight to gain when expecting and why, and postpregnancy weight-loss guidelines

- How much exercise you need in every stage of your life and every trimester, who should not work out during pregnancy, and what activities to avoid
- How diet and lifestyle affect your chances of conceiving a child
- What your partner needs to do to increase his chances of fathering the healthiest child possible
- The nutrients necessary for your well-being—and your baby's—before, during, and after pregnancy; why they matter, how much of them you need, and how to work them into an easy-to-follow eating plan that fits your lifestyle
- Realistic, balanced eating plans, whether you're thinking about having a baby, you're pregnant, or you're breast-feeding; if you want to gain weight, lose some pounds, or stay the same weight to prepare for motherhood
- How diet and lifestyle help you to dodge or manage the complications and discomforts of pregnancy
- Information about your diet and exercise during the "fourth trimester," the months immediately following delivery
- Which vitamins and minerals you need prior to and during pregnancy
- All of the food safety information you need for the well-being of you and your developing child
- More than fifty delicious and nutritious easy-to-prepare recipes and meal ideas, designed to maximize nutrition
- Dozens of resources on a range of topics, including childbirth, breast-feeding, infertility, and food safety

Ultimately, you'll make up your own mind about what to eat before and during pregnancy and after delivery. *Expect the Best* will be there for you every step of the way, gently guiding you in a helpful manner to make the healthiest child possible.

1

Prepregnancy: Starting from a Healthy Place

There's no need to wait for a positive pregnancy test to start working on a healthy lifestyle. When a balanced diet and regular physical activity are part of your everyday routine, your future child will benefit at birth and for a lifetime.

Now is a good time for you, and your partner, to examine what improvements you can make before you try to have a baby. No matter how diligent you are in the pursuit of good health, there's probably room for improvement.

A Plan for a Healthier Pregnancy

You may envision preconception care as nothing more than a single visit to your gynecologist, internal medicine physician, certified nurse-midwife, or nurse practitioner in the months before conception, but health experts see preparing for pregnancy differently. In 2005, the Centers for Disease Control and Prevention came out with recommendations for improving the health of the estimated sixty-three million American women of childbearing age before they conceive, whether it's their first child or their fourth.

For women in their childbearing years who can become pregnant, priming the body for pregnancy is an ongoing pursuit. In fact, your prebaby health and your health between pregnancies should be a high priority with your primary care provider (the doctor you see for yearly physicals and when you get ill). Being ready for pregnancy is considered so important that the American Academy of Pediatrics and the American College of Obstetricians and Gynecologists recommend that your primary care provider and your obstetrician gynecologist (ob-gyn) provide information about preconception care and risk reduction before and between pregnancies at every visit you have with them. You can prompt a discussion about your preconception care with your primary care provider, your dentist, and your registered dietitian by letting them know that you're planning for a child and asking what you should be doing to prepare yourself. Preconception care should be tailored to meet your needs and to account for any chronic conditions you have, such as a weight problem (either too much or too little), high blood pressure, diabetes, or a combination of factors.

The idea of having your body ready for pregnancy makes sense on many levels. More than half of all pregnancies in the United States are unplanned. Taking care of yourself reduces the risk of problems for your unborn baby, especially when pregnancy catches you off guard. Developing babies are highly susceptible to birth defects and other problems during the first eight weeks of pregnancy, when women often do not realize they are expecting or well before they have their first prenatal visit with a healthcare professional.

It's especially important that women seek medical advice prior to conceiving in order to prevent problems with subsequent pregnancies if they've ever had the following problems: a low-birth-weight baby (a child who weighs less than five and a half pounds at birth); a preterm infant (born between the twentieth and thirty-seventh week of pregnancy); a child with a birth defect; or infant death.

A Preconception To-Do List

In addition to having regular medical checkups and a thorough physical examination before conception, a mother-to-be can take several steps to improve her well-being.

Check Your Weight

When you're trying to have a baby, your body weight takes on new meaning. For instance, the right weight makes it easier to get pregnant. That's because either too much or too little body fat interferes with a woman's fertility. There's even some evidence that it might be more difficult for overweight and underweight women to conceive by means of high-tech methods such as in vitro fertilization.

If both you and your partner are overweight, it could take even longer to conceive a child than if only one of you needs to shed some pounds. A 2007 *Human Reproduction* study found that excess body fat interferes with a man's fertility (see chapter 7 for more on this).

In addition to affecting fertility, excess body fat on a woman at the time of conception has been linked to a greater risk for certain birth defects known as structural defects, which include neural tube defects (NTDs). Many NTDs, such as spina bifida, are preventable by consuming adequate folic acid very early in pregnancy. Nevertheless, even folic acid might not protect overweight women from having a pregnancy affected by an NTD. Heart defects and omphalocele, a type of intestinal hernia, are also more likely in infants born to overweight women.

Carrying around extra pounds makes you prone to diabetes before, during, and after pregnancy, which could be problematic for you and your child. Animal and human studies suggest that women with diabetes before pregnancy deliver more babies with structural defects. In addition, women who enter pregnancy overweight tend to stay overweight for the duration of their pregnancy, which increases the likelihood of complications during pregnancy and delivery.

Starting pregnancy at a healthy weight gives your child a much better chance of developing normally. It also helps to lower the risk of the following complications for you during pregnancy:

- High blood pressure
- Gestational diabetes (diabetes during pregnancy)
- Induced labor (which can require more medication to get the job done and which can also lead to a longer labor)
- Cesarean section
- A larger baby who is more difficult to deliver

- A child who scores lower on the Apgar test, which measures a newborn's physical condition at one minute and five minutes after delivery
- Preterm labor and delivery
- A pregnancy that ends in stillbirth (death after the twentieth week of pregnancy)

How will you know what body weight is right for you? You're probably aware that suggested body weight is associated with how tall you are, but you might not know that there is no single weight that's considered the healthiest. Rather, there is a range for each height.

Determining your body mass index (BMI) is the most accurate way to know whether your weight falls within the healthy range. BMI indicates body fat based on a (nonpregnant) adult's height and weight. Measure your height in stocking feet (with no shoes on). For the greatest accuracy, jump on the scale naked, first thing in the morning, after using the bathroom and before eating or drinking. Then consult the chart on pages 12–13 to determine your BMI.

You can also find your BMI with the BMI calculator from the National Heart, Lung, and Blood Institute (NHLBI) at www.nhlbisupport.com/bmi/.

Now that you know where you stand, should you lose weight, put on some pounds, or stay the same? No matter what your goal, you'll need a healthy eating plan to follow. See chapter 3 to create a balanced diet.

Fill the Nutrient Gaps in Your Diet

You may look great and generally feel good, too, but if you're like many American women, you might be marginally deficient in several nutrients that could prevent you from conceiving in tip-top condition, even when your weight is in the healthy range.

The Dietary Guidelines for Americans 2005 (DGA), a joint effort of the U. S. Department of Agriculture and the U.S. Department of Health and Human Services, serve as the blueprint for healthy eating and exercise for Americans over the age of two.

According to the DGA, adults do not get a sufficient amount of the following nutrients in their diet:

- Calcium
- Fiber
- Magnesium
- Vitamin E

- Vitamin C
- Carotenoids, such as beta-carotene (used by the body to make vitamin A)
- Potassium

In addition, women are encouraged to be sure to get the following two nutrients during their childbearing years:

- Iron
- Folic acid

It's important to have adequate levels of these nutrients in your diet before, during, and after pregnancy. For example, dietary iron helps you to maintain the proper iron levels in your body. Iron is critical for transporting oxygen in the body, among other functions. Several studies suggest that iron stores at the time of conception are a strong indicator of your risk for iron-deficiency anemia later in pregnancy, when iron needs increase dramatically. Iron deficiency during pregnancy can increase the risk for preterm delivery. It's difficult to replenish depleted iron stores once pregnancy has begun.

Focus on Folate

Folate, along with its synthetic cousin, folic acid, is not one of the major problem nutrients identified by the Dietary Guidelines for Americans 2005, but it is mentioned as a nutrient to which women in their childbearing years should pay particular attention. Women whose diets fall short of fruits, vegetables, legumes (beans), and fortified grains (and who do not take dietary supplements) might not consume the recommended amounts of folate. Folate and folic acid help to prevent neural tube defects (NTDs) within the first month or so of pregnancy, when the neural tube forms. The neural tube eventually develops into your baby's spine and brain. Women who have had a pregnancy affected by an NTD need about ten times more than the recommended 400 micrograms of folic acid every day very early in their pregnancy. You may require additional folic acid if you're carrying multiple fetuses or have diabetes or epilepsy. Folic acid can prevent miscarriage, along with helping the developing fetus with other important functions. Read up on folic acid and folate in chapter 2.

Body Mass Index																	
	Normal						Overweight					Obese					
BMI	19	20	21	22	23	24	25	26	27	28	29	30	31	32	33	34	35	36
Height (inches)	Body Weight (pounds)																	
58	91	96	100	105	110	115	119	124	129	134	138	143	148	153	158	162	167	172
59	94	99	104	109	114	119	124	128	133	138	143	148	153	158	163	168	173	178
60	97	102	107	112	118	123	128	133	138	143	148	153	158	163	168	174	179	184
61	100	106	111	116	122	127	132	137	143	148	153	158	164	169	174	180	185	190
62	104	109	115	120	126	131	136	142	147	153	158	164	169	175	180	186	191	196
63	107	113	118	124	130	135	141	146	152	158	163	169	175	180	186	191	197	203
64	110	116	122	128	134	140	145	151	157	163	169	174	180	186	192	197	204	209
65	114	120	126	132	138	144	150	156	162	168	174	180	186	192	198	204	210	216
66	118	124	130	136	142	148	155	161	167	173	179	186	192	198	204	210	216	223
67	121	127	134	140	146	153	159	166	172	178	185	191	198	204	211	217	223	230
68	125	131	138	144	151	158	164	171	177	184	190	197	203	210	216	223	230	236
69	128	135	142	149	155	162	169	176	182	189	196	203	209	216	223	230	236	243
70	132	139	146	153	160	167	174	181	188	195	202	209	216	222	229	236	243	250
71	136	143	150	157	165	172	179	186	193	200	208	215	222	229	236	243	250	257
72	140	147	154	162	169	177	184	191	199	206	213	221	228	235	242	250	258	265
73	144	151	159	166	174	182	189	197	204	212	219	227	235	242	250	257	265	272
74	148	155	163	171	179	186	194	202	210	218	225	233	241	249	256	264	272	280
75	152	160	168	176	184	192	200	208	216	224	232	240	248	256	264	272	279	287
76	156	164	172	180	189	197	205	213	221	230	238	246	254	263	271	279	287	295

Body Mass Index																	
	Obese			Extreme Obesity													
BMI	37	38	39	40	41	42	43	44	45	46	47	48	49	50	51	52	53	54
Height (inches)	Body Weight (pounds)																	
58	177	181	186	191	196	201	205	210	215	220	224	229	234	239	244	248	253	258
59	183	188	193	198	203	208	212	217	222	227	232	237	242	247	252	257	262	267
60	189	194	199	204	209	215	220	225	230	235	240	245	250	255	261	266	271	276
61	195	201	206	211	217	222	227	232	238	243	248	254	259	264	269	275	280	285
62	202	207	213	218	224	229	235	240	246	251	256	262	267	273	278	284	289	295
63	208	214	220	225	231	237	242	248	254	259	265	270	278	282	287	293	299	304
64	215	221	227	232	238	244	250	256	262	267	273	279	285	291	296	302	308	314
65	222	228	234	240	246	252	258	264	270	276	282	288	294	300	306	312	318	324
66	229	235	241	247	253	260	266	272	278	284	291	297	303	309	315	322	328	334
67	236	242	249	255	261	268	274	280	287	293	299	306	312	319	325	331	338	344
68	243	249	256	262	269	276	282	289	295	302	308	315	322	328	335	341	348	354
69	250	257	263	270	277	284	291	297	304	311	318	324	331	338	345	351	358	365
70	257	264	271	278	285	292	299	306	313	320	327	334	341	348	355	362	369	376
71	265	272	279	286	293	301	308	315	322	329	338	343	351	358	365	372	379	386
72	272	279	287	294	302	309	316	324	331	338	346	353	361	368	375	383	390	397
73	280	288	295	302	310	318	325	333	340	348	355	363	371	378	386	393	401	408
74	287	295	303	311	319	326	334	342	350	358	365	373	381	389	396	404	412	420
75	295	303	311	319	327	335	343	351	359	367	375	383	391	399	407	415	423	431
76	304	312	320	328	336	344	353	361	369	377	385	394	402	410	418	426	435	443

Although multivitamin and mineral pills are no match for a balanced diet, they are highly beneficial for women in their childbearing years, especially those who don't eat well or who avoid animal products. Multivitamin and mineral pills help to fill any gaps in essential nutrients in your diet.

Dietary supplements are just that, however—supplements. They are missing appreciable amounts of several of the nutrients identified as problematic by the DGA (see page 10), including potassium and calcium as well as the carbohydrate, protein, and fat that are required to produce the energy that fuels all of your bodily functions. Nevertheless, taking a multivitamin pill is a low-risk, relatively low-cost approach to improving the chances of having the healthiest baby possible. Here are some additional reasons to take a daily supplement:

- Taking a multivitamin every day prior to conception reduced the risk of preterm birth by about half in a group of about two thousand women in a study from the University of North Carolina at Chapel Hill.
- Another study from the same university suggests that there is a beneficial relationship between multivitamin use during pregnancy and a 30 to 40 percent reduced risk of neuroblastoma, a tumor of the nervous system. Though relatively rare, according to the American Cancer Society, neuroblastoma is the most common type of cancer in infants and the fourth most common type of cancer in children.

- Women who took multivitamins before and during pregnancy reduced the risk of delivering children with congenital (present at birth) heart defects by 24 percent, according to researchers at the Centers for Disease Control and Prevention. The heart forms in the first trimester of pregnancy, when a woman might not be aware of her pregnancy and might not be getting the nutrients she needs.
- An analysis of forty-one studies suggests a strong link between taking multivitamins before and throughout the first trimester of pregnancy and a reduction in NTDs, heart defects, limb deformities, and cleft palates.

> WORDS OF
> *Motherly Wisdom*
>
> "As soon as we decided to have a baby, I started taking a multivitamin every day. My husband did, too! I've taken vitamins ever since."
> —*Sarah*

Stores offer a slew of multivitamin pills. Look for these qualities when making your choice:

- **No more than 100 percent of the Daily Value (DV) for the nutrients the multi contains, including iron and folic acid.** Since you're eating, you will get nutrients from your food, so there's no need to overdo it with supplements. The DVs are recommended intakes for adults who are neither pregnant nor nursing. They are useful guidelines for women trying to conceive.

- **Fewer than 3,000 International Units of vitamin A, with the majority of it in the form of beta-carotene.** Consuming excessive amounts of vitamin A as retinol (the preformed variety that is often found in dietary supplements and called *vitamin A acetate* or *palmitate*) increases the chances for birth defects in a developing baby. In addition, too much vitamin A from retinol is toxic to the liver and bad for your bones. Beta-carotene, the raw material the body converts to vitamin A, is safer. Supplemental beta-carotene is not known to increase the risk of birth defects.

- **A knockoff of a big-name brand.** Store brands typically cost less and contain the same nutrients as name brands. Stay away from special formulations, such as a women's multivitamin, which tend to cost more and supply nutrients you don't need, including herbs and other botanicals. Herbs and other botanicals add to the cost of multivitamins and have not been proven safe for pregnant women.

- **The U.S. Pharmecopia symbol.** The USP symbol ensures that the supplement has been tested for product safety and quality—that you are getting what you are paying for and that it is dissolving in your body so it can be absorbed.

Get Medical Checkups

It's important to be checked for certain conditions, such as iron-deficiency anemia and diabetes, during your regular preventive health appointments with your primary care physician, nurse practitioner, ob-gyn, or certified nurse-midwife. Regular screening, such as a yearly blood test (often referred to as a complete blood count, or CBC) may turn up problems that you can deal with well before pregnancy. Taking control of medical conditions before pregnancy will produce the healthiest outcomes once you're expecting.

Iron

You may be one of the estimated eight million women of childbearing age with an iron deficiency that's severe enough to cause anemia, and you might not even know it. It's harder to correct iron-deficiency anemia during pregnancy, when the demand for iron skyrockets, so it's beneficial to catch the condition before conception and try to correct it.

Simply testing for iron in your blood may not be enough to determine if you are at risk for iron-deficiency anemia. Have your health-care provider test for ferritin, a reflection of stored iron in the body. Checking your ferritin level is a better way to gauge your chances for iron-deficiency anemia. A low ferritin level in the bloodstream means that you might have the condition.

WORDS OF
Motherly Wisdom

"I had anemia with my first pregnancy, so I was careful about getting enough iron before I got pregnant with my other children."
—Kara

Diabetes

According to the American Diabetes Association, about 54 percent of the U.S. population is at risk for developing diabetes because they have prediabetes: a blood glucose concentration that registers outside the normal range but is not yet elevated enough for a diagnosis of diabetes. Prediabetes can be a sign of what's to come. Elevated blood glucose concentrations now translate into a greater chance for developing gestational diabetes and type 2 diabetes later on. Women with prediabetes and diabetes during pregnancy tend to have more complicated pregnancies, and they often give birth to larger infants who may require a cesarean delivery.

During pregnancy, the extra glucose in your blood can result in your baby's growing too large. Large babies at birth run a greater risk of becoming overweight and developing type 2 diabetes later in life. In addition, when a baby is "fed" extra glucose in utero, the pancreas produces additional insulin, the hormone that helps glucose to gain entry to cells. After delivery, it can be difficult for a child's pancreas to stop making the surplus insulin that was needed before birth, which often results in low blood sugar levels in newborns. Once born, a baby no longer receives surplus glucose from the mother. Yet, the baby's body is still producing too much insulin, which makes for low blood sugar levels.

Jaundice, a buildup of old red blood cells, is also more common in babies delivered by women with diabetes, and these children are more likely to have low supplies of iron in their livers, which can result in iron-deficiency anemia.

It's possible to have prediabetes and not know it, because the condition is often symptom-free. Measuring your glucose level as part of a blood test after fasting is a great way to find out if you're at risk. (A fasting level is obtained after going nine hours without eating.) A normal blood glucose value is below 100 milligrams per deciliter (mg/dl). If you have prediabetes, your fasting blood glucose level will measure between 100 and 125 mg/dl. When the fasting blood glucose level rises to 126 mg/dl or above, you have diabetes.

The good news is that even when your blood glucose level is higher than normal, the chances are that it will drop when you lose weight and exercise regularly. Changing your diet and physical activity for the better significantly delays or prevents the onset of type 2 diabetes. For some people with prediabetes, getting control of a high blood glucose level can reverse the condition and return the glucose level to within a healthy range. For example, losing just ten to fifteen pounds can mean the difference between unhealthy and normal blood glucose concentrations.

A fasting blood glucose level is typically part of the blood test in a complete physical examination, but ask for it anyway, especially if you are overweight and have any of the following risk factors for diabetes:

- High blood pressure
- Low levels of high-density lipoprotein cholesterol (the "good" cholesterol) and elevated triglycerides (fat) in the blood
- A family history of diabetes
- A history of gestational diabetes or giving birth to a baby weighing more than nine pounds
- Belonging to an ethnic group that is at high risk for diabetes: African Americans, Latinos, Native Americans, and Asian Americans/Pacific Islanders

Diagnosis: Diabetes

If you have diabetes, you've got company. According to the Centers
for Disease Control and Prevention, diabetes (type 1 and type 2)
affects about 1.85 million American women ages eighteen to forty-
four. Women with either type of diabetes are three times more likely
than women without diabetes to deliver a baby with a birth defect,
to miscarry, or to have a pregnancy end in infant death. The infants
of women who had diabetes throughout pregnancy are also prone to
higher blood pressure and to becoming overweight in childhood.

Nevertheless, there is good news. Getting control of your glucose
level greatly increases your chances of having a healthy baby. The
American Diabetes Association recommends that you have an A1C
(also known as glycated hemoglobin) level of less than 1 percent
above normal range, which is considered to be 4 to 6 percent, before
you attempt conception. Your A1C concentration reflects the average
of your blood glucose levels for the past few months and provides a
better picture of blood glucose control than any single blood glucose
test. It's important to strive for good blood glucose control at all times
during your childbearing years, since you might not know you're
expecting for two weeks or more after conception occurs, which is a
critical time for a baby's organ development.

Cholesterol and Blood Lipids

Excessive blood cholesterol is not good for your heart and brain, and it
can influence the health of your growing child, too. During pregnancy,
high levels of blood lipids (fats) suppress a substance in the body called
prostacyclin, which results in the narrowing of blood vessels as well as
blood clotting in the vessels that transport oxygen and nutrients to the
womb. Experts say that an expectant mother's elevated blood lipids (such
as cholesterol) can also boost her child's risk of heart disease as an adult.
Elevated cholesterol levels during pregnancy have also been linked to
preeclampsia, a dangerous medical condition marked by elevated blood
pressure and protein in the urine.

According to the NHLBI, people age twenty and older should have
their lipids measured at least once every five years. Request a lipoprotein

profile to get the best idea of where you stand. This blood test is done after you have fasted for at least nine hours. A lipoprotein profile provides information about the following:

- Total cholesterol
- Low-density lipoprotein (LDL) cholesterol, the main source of the cholesterol that contributes to buildup and blockage in the arteries
- High-density lipoprotein (HDL) cholesterol, which helps to keep cholesterol from accumulating in the arteries and blocking the blood flow
- Triglycerides, the fat in the blood that has been linked to heart disease

Compare your lipoprotein profile to the following NHLBI goals for adults:

Total cholesterol: 200 mg/dl or less
LDL cholesterol: 100 mg/dl or less
HDL cholesterol: 40 mg/dl or more
Triglycerides: 150 mg/dl or less

Although your diet, body weight, and physical activity influence blood lipid levels, heredity also plays a role. To reduce blood lipids and keep them in check, follow an eating plan that is low in total and saturated fat. Lose weight, if necessary, to reduce total and LDL cholesterol. Exercise on a regular basis to boost HDL cholesterol and reduce total and LDL cholesterol.

The Thyroid

The thyroid gland produces thyroxine, a hormone that controls the pace of all bodily processes, which are collectively called *metabolism*. When the thyroid is sluggish, a condition called *hypothyroidism*, the thyroxine level falls. As a result, you might feel colder, tire more easily, have drier skin, become forgetful or depressed, and have bouts of constipation. In *hyperthyroidism*, excess thyroxine speeds up the metabolism, causing an array of symptoms such as irritability, increased heart rate, anxiety, weight loss in spite of a good appetite, and irregular menstrual periods.

Hypothyroidism is one of the most common thyroid disorders. About 2 to 3 percent of Americans have pronounced hypothyroidism, and as many as another 15 percent have a milder form that can be symptom-free. Hypothyroidism is more prevalent in women than in men, and it's particularly common in women in their childbearing years. More than half of all people with hypothyroidism are not aware that they have it, according to the American Thyroid Association.

There is no consensus of opinion regarding screening all women for hypothyroidism during pregnancy. However, some physician groups, including the American Association of Clinical Endocrinologists, recommend checking a woman's thyroid function before she conceives or as soon as pregnancy is confirmed. This is especially true for women at high risk for thyroid disease, such as those who have previously been treated for hyperthyroidism or who have a positive family history of thyroid disease.

Testing your thyroid is important. By the end of the first trimester, your child's thyroid will be making its own thyroid hormones. Until then, the baby will be completely dependent on you for the correct balance of compounds that maximize brain development. Babies born to mothers whose bodies don't produce enough of the thyroid hormone thyroxine are prone to shorter attention spans and lower IQ scores as children.

A baby who has started to produce thyroid hormones requires iodine, a mineral that serves as a raw material for thyroid hormones. Your diet supplies the iodine your child needs. See chapter 2 for more about iodine.

Vaccinations

Women in their childbearing years should keep their vaccinations up-to-date. According to the American College of Obstetricians and Gynecologists and the March of Dimes, women should make sure that they are current with the following vaccinations before they try to conceive:

- Tetanus-diphtheria booster
- Measles, mumps, and rubella
- Varicella (chicken pox)
- Human papillomavirus (HPV)
- Meningococcal

Some of these shots are live viruses, which should be avoided during pregnancy. Wait a month after receiving any vaccine to try to conceive.

You may also need the following shots (check with your health-care provider):

- Hepatitis A
- Hepatitis B
- Influenza (flu) vaccine (made from an inactivated virus)
- Pneumococcal
- Rabies

Feeling Blue?

Your emotional well-being is just as important as your physical health. If you have felt sad or hopeless lately or you derive little pleasure in life, you could be depressed. Talk with your doctor about being screened for depression.

Pay a Visit to Your Dentist

An attractive smile is more than a reflection of your mood. Your mouth serves as a gateway to the rest of the body, including germs that can put your pregnancy at risk. Untreated mouth infections are linked to complications for women and their infants.

An analysis of seventeen published scientific articles in the *American Journal of Obstetrics & Gynecology* concluded that there's probably an association between preterm birth or low-birth-weight infants and periodontal disease (PD) in their mothers. PD is a chronic infection of the gums, caused by the bacteria present in plaque, the colorless film that forms on teeth. The most likely culprit is a labor-inducing chemical called *prostaglandin*. Women with severe PD have very high levels of prostaglandin in their mouths.

Gingivitis is the mildest type of PD. It causes red, swollen gums that bleed easily. Gingivitis is usually painless, and it is reversible with professional treatment and vigilant at-home oral hygiene. A normal pregnancy can cause the gums to swell or bleed in a condition called *pregnancy gingivitis*, which often shows up in the second or third month of pregnancy.

WORDS OF
Motherly Wisdom

"I am so glad that my dental hygienist pointed out how important it was to take good care of your mouth prior to pregnancy. I got regular checkups and took care of any problems before I got pregnant."
—*Sarah*

It's important to make every effort to complete any necessary dental work, such as fillings or crowns, before conception. Confirm that you are not pregnant before having dental X-rays and local anesthetic, neither of which is good for the baby. Here are some other dental hygiene tips for mothers-to-be:

- See your dentist immediately if you are having any dental problems, such as bleeding gums, whether you are pregnant or not.
- Brush after every meal, floss at least once a day, and use a fluoride rinse daily.
- If you're at risk for gum disease, have frequent dental visits. Discuss with your dentist how often you should be seen.
- Eat carbohydrate-rich foods, such as bread and crackers, with meals and have sweet desserts soon after, if at all. Consider eating cheese at the end of a meal instead of having cookies, cake, or ice cream. Cheese neutralizes detrimental mouth bacteria, whereas carbohydrates energize them.
- Drink milk. The calcium in milk strengthens the bone in your jaw that helps to hold your teeth in place, and the vitamin D helps your body to absorb the calcium.

Mind Your Medications

Many medications that you use without a second thought are safe for you, but they could have dire consequences for your unborn child, especially during the first trimester when the organs are forming. Illicit drugs, including marijuana and cocaine, could also be harmful.

Excessive levels of vitamin A in acne medications such as Accutane (isotretinoin) should be avoided by women who are pregnant or who may become pregnant because of the risk of miscarriage and birth defects. It is extremely important for sexually active women who could become pregnant and who take vitamin A–based acne medications to use an effective method of birth control. Women of childbearing age who take these medications are advised to undergo monthly pregnancy tests to make sure they are not pregnant.

Even seemingly harmless over-the-counter medications, such as common pain relievers, can be detrimental before and during pregnancy. A *British Medical Journal* study found a connection between miscarriage and taking aspirin, ibuprofen, or other nonsteroidal anti-inflammatory drugs around the time of conception or in early pregnancy. The link was stronger when women took those medications for more than one week. Acetaminophen, however, was not associated with greater miscarriage risk. Taking aspirin in the third trimester is linked to excessive bleeding in the mother and the baby at delivery. This doesn't mean that all medications for chronic conditions are off-limits during pregnancy. For example, women with an underactive thyroid must continue on levothyroxine throughout pregnancy to ensure proper neurological development in their children. The dose will probably change once you conceive, however.

Talk with your doctor and your pharmacist about what medications are safe when you're trying to conceive, when you are pregnant, or when you're nursing. You might think that because herbs and other dietary supplements are made from plants, they're okay to take, but that's not necessarily true. There's no guarantee that herbal products are safe, especially during pregnancy. Herbal products are not regulated by the Food and Drug Administration, the government organization that oversees drug safety. This means that many herbs and botanicals do not have to adhere to the same standards for safety and effectiveness that drugs do. In addition, because herbs and botanicals are not regulated, you can't always be sure of what you are buying. That's why it's best to avoid herbs and botanical supplements altogether when you're trying to conceive or are pregnant or nursing.

Herbal Tea Alert

Although herbal teas are caffeine-free, there is simply too little scientific data about the safety of teas made from many herbs. The chances are that the types of herbal teas in filtered bags that are available on supermarket shelves, such as chamomile and peppermint, are safe in reasonable amounts. Avoid herbal teas that are not commercially produced, however. For more information about herbal teas and dietary supplements, visit the Natural Medicines Database at www.therapeuticresearch.com. Click on the Natural Medicines Comprehensive Database, which provides information for consumers.

Assess Alcohol Intake

No alcohol intake is the recommendation during pregnancy, but how about when you're trying to conceive? It seems to be okay to enjoy a glass of wine or a cocktail when you think you're not pregnant. Nevertheless, experts, including the March of Dimes and the Centers for Disease Control and Prevention, say otherwise. They contend that drinking alcohol and trying to conceive do not mix.

Although moderate drinking—defined as no more than one drink per day for women—is often touted as beneficial to your health when you're not pregnant or nursing, it can make it more difficult to conceive a child. You could also be pregnant and not know it. Alcohol is never good for a developing baby, but it's particularly problematic during the first trimester. When you drink, your baby drinks, too. Alcohol passes easily and swiftly through the placenta to your child. An unborn baby's body cannot process alcohol as swiftly as an adult's body can. This means that your child's blood alcohol concentration will be higher than yours and will stay elevated longer.

Alcohol can cause irreversible harm even before you realize you're expecting, by depriving the baby of the oxygen and nutrients that are required for the development of every organ.

Heavy drinking during pregnancy—including the regular consumption of beer, wine, or spirits (the vodka used in martinis or the gin in a gin and tonic, for example)—increases the risk of mental retardation, learning disabilities, birth defects, and emotional and behavioral problems, such as those included in fetal alcohol syndrome (FAS).

FAS is the leading preventable cause of mental retardation in the United States. FAS tends to be associated with regular heavy drinking during pregnancy, but even moderate alcohol intake has been linked to impaired fetal growth and lower Apgar scores. Newborns are given the Apgar test at one minute and five minutes after delivery to measure their physical condition and their need for medical attention.

The Definition of a Drink

The size of "a drink" might be smaller than you think. Twelve ounces of regular beer, five ounces of wine, or one and a half ounces of 80-proof distilled spirits (such as rum, vodka, or whiskey) is considered a drink.

It's clear that even some drinking of alcohol during pregnancy is dangerous. A 2002 study found that fourteen-year-old children whose mothers had as little as one drink a week were significantly shorter and more likely to be underweight than children of women who did not drink at all. A 2001 *Pediatrics* study found that six- and seven-year-old children of mothers who sipped just one drink a week during pregnancy were more likely than children of nondrinkers to have behavior problems, such as aggressive and delinquent behaviors.

Consuming alcohol during pregnancy also increases the risk of miscarriage, low birth weight (less than five and a half pounds), and stillbirth. A 2002 Danish study found that women who consumed five or more drinks a week were three times more likely to have a stillborn baby than women who had less than one drink a week.

If you took an occasional drink before you knew you were pregnant, the chances are that no harm was done. Discuss any concerns you have with your doctor or nurse-midwife.

Consider Caffeine Intake

As anyone with a caffeine habit knows, caffeine is a stimulant that increases alertness.

Reasonable amounts of caffeine, which are considered to be less than 200 milligrams (mg) a day, probably have little effect on fertility, but consuming 500 mg or more—about the amount found in sixteen ounces of regular Starbucks coffee or two cans of diet cola—every day might delay conception and cause other problems with a pregnancy. Perhaps you should kick your caffeine cravings when you want to conceive.

The major source of caffeine is coffee, but it can also be found in tea, soft drinks, energy drinks, candy, gum, ice cream, and some medications. See chapter 2 to tally your daily caffeine intake and see if you should cut down.

What to Do If You Have Difficulty Getting Pregnant

Perhaps you're doing everything you should to get pregnant, but to no avail. If you've been trying to conceive (that is, having unprotected intercourse) for at least twelve months or you are older than thirty-five and have been trying for at least six months, you could be experiencing infertility (see chapter 7 for the causes of infertility as well as how diet and lifestyle affect the chances of conception).

Stop Smoking

Smoking jeopardizes your health and makes you less able to tolerate the rigors of pregnancy. It can also put a damper on fertility. Studies show that women who smoke often have more trouble conceiving than non-smokers do.

Smoking during pregnancy does irreparable harm to the baby. Cigarette smoke contains thousands of chemicals in addition to nicotine. Although it's uncertain exactly which chemicals harm a developing fetus, one thing is certain: nicotine and carbon monoxide reduce the supply of oxygen your child needs to grow and develop properly. This could be why smoking cigarettes increases the risk of a smaller baby, a preterm baby, and infant death. Smoking during pregnancy is also linked to mental retardation and nicotine addiction in children. Some studies have shown that smoking increases the risk of facial deformities, such as cleft palate.

According to the U.S. Public Health Service, if all pregnant women in the United States stopped smoking, there would be an estimated 11 percent reduction in stillbirths and a 5 percent reduction in newborn deaths. If you're a smoker who is planning to quit once you're pregnant, don't wait till then. It's unwise to put off kicking the cigarette habit. Only about 20 percent of women successfully give up cigarettes during pregnancy, so start now. It often takes several attempts before you give up cigarettes for good.

If you quit smoking but your partner does not, your baby's growth and birth weight can still be affected by your exposure to secondhand smoke during pregnancy. Avoid exposure to other people's smoke as much as possible in order to limit harm to your child. Encourage your partner to quit or at least not to smoke when you're around. You're more likely to stay off cigarettes when you get support from your friends and your family.

Don't plan on lighting up again once the baby is born. Babies who are exposed to secondhand smoke suffer more than other babies from lower-respiratory illnesses (such as bronchitis and pneumonia), asthma, and ear infections, and they run a greater risk of sudden infant death syndrome.

Consider Safety Issues

When you're trying to conceive, it's important to educate yourself about the foods that could cause health problems later on when you're expecting or nursing, including certain seafood, undercooked meat and raw fish, and contaminated water. There are many safety issues to consider when you're preparing for pregnancy (see chapter 6 for more information on what to avoid).

Move Often

You know the many benefits of exercise, so perhaps you're active nearly every day of the week. Maybe you're too tired or too busy, or working out is boring. Whatever the case, it pays to know how exercise influences your future child's health.

The following benefits of exercise may motivate you to work out on a regular basis:

- Easier weight control
- Less stress, depression, and anxiety
- A reduced risk of colon cancer
- A stronger heart and a lower pulse rate
- Better muscle tone, more flexible joints, and stronger bones
- A reduced risk of type 2 diabetes and better management of blood glucose levels in type 1 and type 2 diabetes
- Lower levels of total and LDL (low-density lipoprotein) cholesterol and improved levels of HDL (high-density lipoprotein) cholesterol in the bloodstream
- Healthy blood pressure
- Improved circulation
- Clearer thinking

Research suggests that regular physical activity is good for your baby, too. A study published in the *Maternal and Child Health Journal* found that physically active women had a 30 to 50 percent lower risk for pregnancies affected by neural tube defects even when they did not take multivitamins prior to conception and regardless of their weight. In addition, researchers at the University of Washington who surveyed 688 mothers found that those who performed the most vigorous exercise during the year before pregnancy were 81 percent less likely to develop gestational diabetes—a condition linked to abnormally large babies and difficult labor—than their sedentary peers were; moderate exercisers had a 59 percent lower risk. Furthermore, the benefit held up even when the women were overweight.

How much exercise is enough to reap the health benefits? According to the DGA, adults require a minimum of thirty minutes of exercise on most days for weight maintenance (provided that calorie intake is equivalent to calories burned); sixty minutes to manage body weight and prevent gradual weight gain; and sixty to ninety minutes to maintain weight loss.

It's harder to stick with a fitness regimen than it is to start one: witness the millions of people who join gyms every year (usually in January!) only to go for a few weeks and then never go again. Maintaining an exercise regimen can be tough; maintaining an active lifestyle is often easier. Here are some tips for making physical activity part of your everyday life. Check with your doctor before beginning any exercise program.

- **Break it down**. Combining short bouts of exercise during the day can be beneficial. For example, park your car at least a ten-minute walk away from your destination, instantly guaranteeing twenty minutes of exercise; add another ten-minute walk at lunchtime, and you've got thirty minutes covered. Invest in a pedometer and work your way up to taking ten thousand steps every day, as long as your doctor, nurse practitioner, or certified nurse-midwife says it's okay.
- **Schedule exercise**. Treat working out like an important client who should not be left waiting.
- **Keep a log**. Write down your activities to see how often you exercise. Aim for at least three days a week to start, and work up to a minimum of five.
- **Get support**. Enlist a workout buddy, such as your spouse, partner, friend, or coworker; join a walking group; or take an exercise class.
- **Have an alternate plan**. Keep exercise videos on hand for when inclement weather keeps you indoors. Consider investing in a treadmill or a stationary bike for inside exercise, too. Walk with a few friends; then if one friend cancels, you'll still have other companions to motivate you.

- **Shake it up**. Boredom can spell doom for your exercise routine. Pick at least two activities, such as walking, Pilates, or yoga, and alternate them. Include weight training twice a week for stronger bones, toned muscles, and a more efficient metabolism.

Pregnancy Takes Preparation

Now that you've made it through this information-packed chapter, you have a better understanding of what you and your partner should do to shape up before you try to have a baby, including achieving and maintaining a healthy weight, getting a checkup from your health-care provider, and exercising regularly. Now, it's time to put healthy eating into practice. Chapter 2 builds your nutrition knowledge, focusing on the role that many important nutrients play in having a healthy baby, even well before conception.

2

Great Expectations: How Eating the Right Food Is Good for You and Your Baby

In chapter 1, you learned how your lifestyle and overall health can influence the chances of conceiving and delivering the healthiest child possible. Whether you're waiting to conceive or you're already expecting, there's a good chance you'll need a diet makeover.

You're not alone in this; many women enter pregnancy with eating patterns that lack the nutrients that are required to nourish a baby's growth and development. Improving your diet now can lessen the risk for complications during pregnancy and reduce the risk of chronic conditions (such as obesity, diabetes, and heart disease) in your child later in life.

Every nutrient that's important to you as a healthy adult is critical for your baby's growth. However, certain nutrients are even more important during pregnancy: carbohydrates, protein, and fat.

Carbohydrates

Carbohydrates, a source of much-needed energy for your and your baby's brain, are found in milk, fruits, vegetables, legumes (beans), breads, grains, cookies, and candy. Eating enough carbohydrates also prevents your body from breaking down protein for its calories. This allows protein to perform its important duties, which include supporting your baby's rapid growth and development.

With the exception of products that also contain fiber, each form of carbohydrate provides 4 calories per gram. Yet all carbohydrates are not created equal. The simple sugars, such as the carbohydrate that is found in table sugar and in high-fructose corn syrup, are not as desirable from a health standpoint as the complex carbohydrates, which include starch and fiber.

Whether the source of the carbohydrate is whole-grain bread or a candy bar, the body converts the carbohydrate into glucose, the fuel that makes cells run. Why is there so much scorn for sugar, then? Perhaps it is because of the company it keeps. Most sugary food—cookies, cake, and candy—is also high in fat and packed with calories that can contribute to an unhealthy weight. Even fat-free sugar-filled foods, such as jelly beans, provide calories and little nutrition. Some sugar-laden foods, such as certain breakfast cereals, have more calories than their counterparts with no added sugar. Naturally sweet foods, like fruit, are better for you because they also supply nutrients such as fiber, vitamins, minerals, and water.

Health experts suggest that you consume the bulk of your carbohydrates from foods that are rich in complex carbohydrates. Starch and other complex carbohydrates take longer to digest, so they provide a slower and steadier energy release into the bloodstream. When you eat simple sugars, the carbohydrate is more readily absorbed, producing a sugar rush that is typically followed by an energy lull. In addition, complex carbohydrates are almost always found in conjunction with other nutrients that benefit you at all stages of life. Foods that are rich in complex carbohydrates include breads, cereals, rice, pasta, vegetables, and beans.

Your carbohydrate needs are determined by your daily calorie requirements: 45 to 65 percent of your total calories should come from carbohydrates. For example, you need 202 to 293 grams of carbohydrates a day on an 1,800-calorie diet; 248 to 358 grams on a 2,200-calorie diet; and 281 to 406 grams on a 2,500-calorie diet. There's no need to tally your total carbohydrate intake, but just for the record, the bare minimum is 130

Artificial Sweeteners and Pregnancy: A Good Match?

Generally speaking, it's safe to use sweeteners such as sucralose (Splenda) and aspartame (such as Equal) during pregnancy and nursing. Saccharin is a concern, however, because it is capable of crossing the placenta and lingering in your baby's tissues. Pregnancy is no time to cut calories, so if you're going overboard on sugar substitutes you may need to question your motives; it might be just fine to use sugar or honey sparingly. Also, keep in mind that foods made with sugar substitutes are not necessarily calorie-free. Nor, in the case of diet soft drinks, do they provide appreciable levels of essential nutrients for pregnancy.

---

grams a day when you are not pregnant, 175 grams a day when you are pregnant, and 210 grams a day when you are nursing. Low-carbohydrate diets can leave you feeling fatigued, because carbohydrate is the brain's, and the body's, preferred energy source.

Even when you try your hardest to limit sugar by avoiding sweet treats, it creeps in through processed foods. For example, ketchup, pasta sauce, and bread often contain added sugar in one form or another. Scan the following list of sugar's aliases and avoid them as much as you can:

Sucrose	Corn sweeteners
Fructose	Honey
Glucose	Brown sugar
Dextrose	Raw sugar
Turbinado sugar	Crystal dextrose
Corn syrup	Sorghum syrup
Corn syrup solids	Maple syrup
High-fructose corn syrup	Evaporated cane juice

Balancing healthy foods with your desire for something sweet is challenging, especially when you're craving sugar. Here's how to satisfy your sweet tooth and work in nutrients, too:

- Prepare flavored milk using eight ounces of low-fat plain milk and a teaspoon or two of chocolate, strawberry, or vanilla syrup. Serve warm, if desired.

- Skip store-bought flavored yogurt in favor of mixing eight ounces of plain low-fat yogurt with a teaspoon of low-sugar fruit preserves, honey, or molasses, or add fresh or frozen fruit.
- Purchase low-sugar cereals, like Cheerios, and plain oatmeal, and add fresh or dried fruit for sweetness. Mix higher-sugar cereals with low-sugar, higher-fiber varieties to cut sugar consumption.
- Snack on whole-grain graham crackers and fig bars instead of chocolate chip and cream-filled sandwich cookies.
- Use a quarter less sugar in quick bread and muffin recipes.
- Do not keep tempting sweets in the house.

Dietary Fiber

Fiber contributes no calories (energy) to your diet because your body is largely incapable of digesting it. Nevertheless, it is important for a number of reasons.

First, it's useful for alleviating constipation, which is a common side effect of pregnancy. Constipation can also occur when you take large doses of supplemental iron. Fiber softens stools and adds bulk, making stools easier to pass. Avoiding constipation helps you to avoid hemorrhoids, which result from straining to move your bowels.

Second, fiber helps to keep you fuller longer, which is beneficial when you're trying to control your weight before pregnancy and after delivery. Third, fiber plays a role in maintaining blood cholesterol level and blood glucose concentration within normal ranges.

Fiber requirements relate to calorie quotas, and they change just slightly with impending motherhood. Nonpregnant women need 25 grams of fiber daily, pregnant women need 28 grams, and nursing women need 29 grams. Fiber absorbs many times its weight in fluid, so it's important to consume a sufficient amount of fluid (water, milk, and juice) each day to keep your digestive tract in working order (see "Fluids" on page 40 for the proper amounts).

Look under "Dietary Fiber" on the nutrient facts panel of food labels for the fiber content of packaged foods. Many foods, such as fruits and vegetables, lack labels, so refer to the following list for their fiber levels.

BEST FOOD SOURCES

Food	Fiber (grams)
Navy beans, cooked, ½ cup	10
Lentils, cooked, ½ cup	8
Black beans, cooked, ½ cup	8
Garbanzo beans, cooked, ½ cup	6
Apple, 1 medium, with skin	4
Strawberries, 1 cup	4
Potato, 1 medium, baked, with skin	4
Sweet potato, 1 medium, flesh only	4
Broccoli, cooked, 1 cup	4
Pasta, whole wheat, cooked, 1 cup	4
Oatmeal, instant, 1 packet	3
Orange, 1 medium	3
Banana, 1 medium	3
Pear, 1 medium, with skin	3

Protein

Protein is the structural component of every part of your body and your baby's body. Pregnant women need dietary protein to support the production of new cells, enzymes, and the hormones that regulate life. Adequate protein during pregnancy helps your baby to grow fully; to develop hair, fingernails, skin, and organs; and to achieve a healthy birth weight. Protein also plays a role in keeping fluid balance in check. Fluid balance is central to preventing pregnancy swelling and maintaining normal blood pressure.

The proteins that are found in your body, such as in your cells and your hormones, are constructed from a series of building blocks called *amino acids*. Amino acids are assembled in particular sequences, depending on the bodily protein. Although protein supplies 4 calories per gram, the body needs food protein primarily for the amino acids it contains. The nitrogen that food protein provides is important, too; nitrogen is central to cell growth and repair.

Both quantity and quality count in fulfilling protein needs. Animal and plant foods provide amino acids, but the protein in animal foods—such as beef, pork, eggs, milk, seafood, and poultry—is different from nearly all plant protein. Animal foods are rich in all of the amino acids that the body cannot make on its own—indispensable amino acids (IAAs)—and must obtain from food. Eggs are particularly prized for their protein quality, because they contain 100 percent of all the IAAs. In fact, the protein quality of all other foods is judged against the levels of IAAs in eggs.

Though nutritious, plant foods, such as most legumes and all grains, lack adequate amounts of one or more of the IAAs. Unlike animal products, no single plant food, with the exception of soy, contains all of the IAAs. Women who avoid or eat few animal foods should aim to include an array of protein-rich plant products such as tofu, soy beverages, and edamame (fresh soybeans) as part of a balanced diet in order to get the right mix of amino acids every day, particularly during pregnancy and nursing. If you are a vegan (that is, you avoid all animal foods, including milk and eggs, from your diet), consult a registered dietitian for help in planning a diet that meets your needs.

Pregnant, nursing, or neither, your protein needs are related to your ideal body weight. You need 0.36 grams of protein per pound per day—about 49 grams for a 135-pound woman—when not pregnant. Starting with the second trimester of your pregnancy, your protein needs increase to 0.5 grams per pound of your prepregnant ideal body weight plus an additional 25 grams, for a total of about 93 grams for a 135-pound woman. If you're having twins, you need an additional 25 grams of protein a day, starting as soon as you find out that you're expecting—about 118 grams of protein a day for a 135-pound woman.

Protein does not come in prenatal vitamins pills or regular multivitamin pills, so plan on filling your daily quota with food. Refer to the following list to see whether your protein intake is up to par.

BEST FOOD SOURCES

Food	Protein (grams)
Chicken breast, skinless, 3 ounces, cooked	26
Pork tenderloin, 3 ounces, roasted	22
Beef, 95% lean, 3 ounces, roasted	22
Salmon, Atlantic, 3 ounces, roasted	22
Tuna, light, canned, drained, 3 ounces	22
Cottage cheese, low-fat, ½ cup	14
Yogurt, plain, low-fat, 1 cup	13
Yogurt, fruit-flavored, low-fat, 1 cup	11
Tofu, raw, ½ cup	10

Food	Protein (grams)
Peanut butter, 2 tablespoons	9
Quinoa, cooked, 1 cup	8
Milk, whole, 1 cup	8
Milk, 1% low-fat, 1 cup	8
Lentils, cooked, ½ cup	8
Black beans, canned, drained, ½ cup	7
Cheddar cheese, 1 ounce	7
Soy beverage, 1 cup	7
Egg, 1 large, cooked any way	6
Pistachios, 1 ounce	6
Garbanzo beans, canned, drained, ½ cup	6
Almond butter, 2 tablespoons	5

Fat

Fat is a three-letter word, but it might as well be a curse, for all the respect it gets. Fat serves up more than twice the calories (9 per gram) of carbohydrates or protein, which is why many women take great pains to shun it. Nevertheless, fat is an essential nutrient to include in a balanced eating plan, whether you are pregnant, planning on becoming pregnant, or nursing a baby. Quality counts, however.

The body requires fat for a couple of reasons. First, fat provides energy. In fact, it would be very difficult to satisfy your calorie needs without fat, and it would certainly be hard to stay healthy. That's because some types of fat supply essential fatty acids (EFAs), compounds that are central to your health and to your child's development. The body cannot produce EFAs—linoleic acid and alpha-linolenic acid—so it must derive them from food. (Infants get EFAs from breast milk and from infant formula.) Second, fat ferries vitamins A, D, E, and K—known as the fat-soluble vitamins—around the body, getting them to where they need to go and fostering their absorption and storage.

Good and Bad Fat

The fat in foods is categorized as *saturated* and *unsaturated*. The majority of another type of fat in the typical American diet, *trans fat*, is man-made. Foods often contain a mixture of fat types, which are listed on the nutrient facts panel of food products.

Animal foods, such as fatty meats and full-fat dairy foods like cheese, ice cream, and whole milk, supply most of the saturated fat that is consumed in the typical American diet. Coconut oil, palm oil, palm kernel oil, and cocoa butter, which are all used widely in packaged foods such as sweets and crackers, are highly saturated fats, too.

Saturated fat is scorned for its role in heart disease. Eating too much saturated fat contributes to clogged arteries, which block blood flow and increase the risk of heart attack and stroke. Pregnant or not, you don't need any saturated fat in your diet because your body produces all that it requires. Nevertheless, there's no need to completely avoid foods with saturated fat in the name of good health. In fact, foods like meat and cheese contain protein, vitamins, and minerals that are vital to a growing baby and a healthy mother.

Trace amounts of naturally occurring trans fat can be found in fatty meats and full-fat dairy foods, but the majority of the trans fat in our food supply is the result of hydrogenation, a process that creates a firmer, tastier product from unsaturated fats. Hydrogenation increases the stability of unsaturated fat, making it ideal to use in processed foods, which require fats with a long shelf life to prevent spoilage. This man-made trans fat is found in margarine, shortening, french fries and other fast foods, cookies, crackers, granola bars, and microwave popcorn. It is bad for the body.

Like saturated fat, trans fat contributes to clogged arteries, and it has been linked to certain cancers. There is no dietary requirement for trans fat, but it's nearly impossible to avoid it completely. Processed products are required to list trans fat content on the food label. There's a hitch, however. A serving of a processed food can contain some trans fat even when the level of trans fat listed is zero ("trans-free"). That's because it's permissible by law to list the trans fat content of a serving of food as zero if it has up to half a gram. Limit trans fat intake with a balanced eating plan that includes minimally processed foods. Use only small amounts of tub margarine or trans fat–free tub margarine, if you must; canola oil and olive oil are preferable for cooking and flavoring foods. Look for the term *partially hydrogenated* in the ingredients list; it lets you know that the product contains trans fat. Experts recommend a limit of 2 grams of trans fat a day for most people, so just a few servings of "trans-free" foods can really add up.

Unsaturated fats are desirable because they are considered heart-healthy. Monounsaturated fat is the primary fat in olive oil, canola oil, sesame oil, avocados, almonds, cashews, pistachios, peanuts, and peanut butter. Polyunsaturated fat is found in corn oil, cottonseed oil, safflower oil, sunflower seeds, flaxseed, and seafood.

Daily fat needs are tied to calorie intake; 20 to 35 percent of your calories should come from fat. There is no need to count fat grams, but it helps to have an idea of your total fat allowance for the day, especially when you are reading food labels. If you're eating 1,800 calories, stick with 40 to 70 grams of fat for the day; for 2,200 calories a day, aim for 49 to 86 grams; and for 2,500 calories, aim for 56 to 97 grams. More than two-thirds of the fat you consume should be unsaturated.

Fish and Fat

Seafood is an excellent source of beneficial fat. Fish and shellfish supply omega-3 fats, which are unsaturated fats that are particularly good for your heart. One omega-3 fat, docosahexaenoic acid (DHA), is central to your child's brain development during pregnancy, nursing, and the first few years of life.

DHA is the dominant fat found in the brain. It's part of every brain cell your child has or will have. Research shows that DHA helps to build your baby's brain, particularly from about the twenty-fourth week of pregnancy, the time when your child's brain is developing at breakneck speed and is hoarding DHA. Preterm babies miss out on the chance to maximize their DHA stores, however.

DHA also contributes to your child's vision by accumulating in the retina, located at the back of each eye. The retina has been called the window to the world because it's involved in registering what you see and transmitting the images to the brain for processing.

As long as your DHA intake is adequate, your child will get the necessary amount from you during pregnancy and nursing. (Most infant formulas also contain DHA.) Many women do not get enough DHA, however. A 2008 *American Journal of Clinical Nutrition* article suggests that some pregnant women are deficient in DHA. Pregnant and nursing women need 200 to 300 mg of DHA daily, but the average intake is only 54 mg a day.

Fish provides you with preformed DHA, the type your body prefers. Adults and children of all ages can convert alpha-linolenic acid—the essential fat found in walnuts, flaxseeds, and other foods—to DHA, but only an estimated 10 percent is actually formed into DHA. Seafood is an easy-to-prepare food that is rich in preformed DHA, protein, vitamins, and minerals and relatively low in total and saturated fat (see chapter 6 for more on seafood).

Preformed DHA is found naturally in seafood. It's also added to dietary supplements and fortified foods. Rely on seafood, fortified foods, and supplements for this important nutrient, like the ones listed below. The fortified foods and dietary supplements in the following list contain an algae-based source of DHA that's free from potential contamination from mercury and other harmful substances.

BEST FOOD SOURCES

Food	DHA (mg)
Salmon, coho, farmed, 3 ounces, cooked	740
Expecta Lipil, 1 pill	200
Gold Circle Farms DHA Omega-3 Eggs, 1 large	150
Blue crab, 3 ounces, cooked	196
Tuna, light, canned, drained, 3 ounces*	190
Catfish, 3 ounces, cooked	116
Oh Mama! bars, 1 bar	115
Bellybars, all flavors, 1 bar	50
Bellybar Chews, all flavors 1 chew	50
Eggland's Best Eggs, 1 large**, cooked any way	50
Cabot 50% Reduced Fat Cheddar Cheese, 1 ounce	32
Bellybar Shakes, 8 ounces	32
Silk Soymilk Plus Omega-3 DHA	32
Horizon Organic Milk Plus DHA Omega-3, 8 ounces	32
Rachel's Wickedly Delicious Yogurt, 8 ounces	32

*You may have heard about tuna and high mercury levels. Canned light tuna is considered acceptable for women in their childbearing years because it's from a smaller species of fish. Canned white tuna is from a larger species of fish, so it's possible that it contains more mercury.

**Supplies 100 mg of omega-3 fats; 50 mg are DHA.

Fluids

You know that water is essential, but do you consider it a nutrient? Water ranks right up there with carbohydrates, protein, fat, and the dozens of other nutrients your body needs. You might say that water is the most essential part of your diet, given the fact that without water, you'd survive just a few days.

Water keeps your body temperature in the normal range for good health. It's part of the transportation system that carries nutrients and waste around, and out of, the body. Water moistens bodily tissues, keeping them in good working condition, and it cushions and protects your developing baby. Water also serves as the basis of breast milk.

Before you conceive, you need about nine (eight-ounce) cups of fluid, including plain water, a day. Pregnant women require about ten cups of fluid every day, and nursing women need about thirteen cups.

Although plain water is preferable, if it's not your beverage of choice, that doesn't necessarily mean that you're low on fluid. Coffee, tea, milk, juice, and carbonated soft drinks count toward your quota, too. Fruits and vegetables are brimming with water and also provide fiber, vitamins, and minerals. Don't overdo it on calorie-containing beverages, such as carbonated soft drinks, however. Too many soft drinks can cause weight gain and take the place of other, more nutritious beverages.

Caffeine

Caffeine is a stimulant that slightly increases blood pressure and heart rate. It is capable of crossing the placenta, and there is some evidence that caffeine can increase fetal heart rate and affect breathing patterns. However, it's unclear whether those changes hurt a developing child.

Most experts agree that small amounts of caffeine (about one small cup of coffee a day) seem to be safe during pregnancy, but the safety of more caffeine during pregnancy is questionable. (Keep in mind that a coffee *mug* is larger than a 1-cup measure.) Higher caffeine consumption can increase the risk of miscarriage, low birth weight, and other problems. A 2003 Danish study published in the *British Medical Journal* suggests that women who drink four or more cups of coffee a day may be at increased risk of having a stillborn baby.

A 2008 study in the *American Journal of Obstetrics and Gynecology* concluded that consuming 200 mg or more of caffeine on a daily basis increased the risk of miscarriage in a group of more than one thousand pregnant women. The higher chance for miscarriage was attributed to caffeine, rather than just coffee; caffeine from noncoffee sources such as soft drinks, tea, and hot chocolate showed a similar risk of miscarriage. The study was so well regarded by health professionals that it prompted the March of Dimes to decrease the recommended daily caffeine limit for pregnant women from

300 to 200 mg a day or less. However, another 2008 study, published in *Epidemiology*, found no risk of miscarriage in a group of women consuming up to 350 mg of caffeine a day. Given the evidence, it probably pays for pregnant women to limit caffeine consumption.

The effects of caffeine on conception is covered in chapter 1.

According to the American Academy of Pediatrics, it's safe for women to consume caffeine while breast-feeding. Remember, however, that even a small amount of caffeine permeates breast milk. Drinking more than two eight-ounce cups of coffee a day (or ingesting the equivalent of any product that contains caffeine) could make for an irritable infant or one who has trouble sleeping.

Coffee is the primary caffeine source, but caffeine shows up in many other foods, too. Most caffeine-laden foods and beverages don't divulge the content on their labels. Rely on the following list to calculate the amount of caffeine in your beverages and food and keep it under the recommended 200 mg a day when you're pregnant.

> WORDS OF
> *Motherly Wisdom*
>
> "Giving up caffeine completely wasn't working for me when I was pregnant with my third child. I had one cup of coffee a day, and it really helped me deal with my other two children!"
> —Meghan

Product	Caffeine (mg)
Coffee	
Starbucks Brewed Coffee (Grande), 16 ounces	330
Einstein Bros. regular coffee, 16 ounces	300
Starbucks Double Shot on Ice, 16 ounces	225
Starbucks Iced Brewed Coffee, 16 ounces	190
Starbucks Cappuccino, 16 ounces	150
Starbucks Frappuccino Blended Coffee Beverages, 16 ounces	110–145
Einstein Bros. Espresso, 1 shot	100
Coffee, generic brewed, 8 ounces	95
Starbucks Espresso, solio, 1 ounce	75
Coffee, generic decaffeinated, 8 ounces	5
Espresso, generic decaffeinated, 1 ounce	0

Product	**Caffeine (mg)**
Tea	
Starbucks Tazo Green Tea Latte (Grande), 16 ounces	80
Tea, black, brewed, 8 ounces	47
Snapple, Lemon (regular and diet versions), 16 ounces	42
Tea, instant powdered, unsweetened, 12 ounces	39
Arizona Iced Tea, black, 20 ounces	31
Tea, green, brewed, 8 ounces	25
Snapple, Just Plain Unsweetened, 16 ounces	18
Arizona Iced Tea, green, 16 ounces	15
Nestea Cool, 12 ounces	11
Snapple, Kiwi Teawi, 16 ounces	10
Lipton, Ready to Drink, 12 ounces	7
Tea, black, brewed, decaffeinated, 8 ounces	2
Soft Drinks	
Jolt Cola, 12 ounces	72
Mountain Dew MDX, regular or diet, 12 ounces	71
Coke Blak, 12 ounces	69
Code Red, regular or diet, 12 ounces	54
Mountain Dew, regular or diet, 12 ounces	54
Pepsi One, 12 ounces	54
Mello Yellow, 12 ounces	53
Diet Coke, 12 ounces	47
TAB, 12 ounces	47
Dr Pepper, regular or diet, 12 ounces	41
Pepsi, 12 ounces	38
Pepsi Twist, 12 ounces	38
Pepsi Wild Cherry, regular or diet, 12 ounces	38
Diet Pepsi, 12 ounces	36
Pepsi Twist diet, 12 ounces	36
Coca-Cola Classic, 12 ounces	35
Barq's Diet Root Beer, 12 ounces	23
Barq's Root Beer, 12 ounces	23
7-Up, regular or diet, 12 ounces	0
Fanta, all flavors, 12 ounces	0

(continued)

Product	Caffeine (mg)
	(continued)
Fresca, all flavors, 12 ounces	0
Mug Root Beer, regular or diet, 12 ounces	0
Sierra Mist, regular or sugar-free, 12 ounces	0
Sprite, regular or diet, 12 ounces	0
Energy Drinks	
Spike Shooter, 8.4 ounces	300
Monster Energy, 16 ounces	160
Rip It, Chic, 8 ounces	150
Full Throttle, 16 ounces	144
Tab Energy, 10.5 ounces	95
SoBe No Fear, 8 ounces	87
SoBe Adrenaline Rush, regular and sugar-free, 8.3 ounces	76
Red Bull, 8.3 ounces	76
Red Bull, sugar-free, 8.3 ounces	75
Glacéau Vitamin Water Energy Citrus, 20 ounces	50
Aquafina Alive Energize, 8 ounces	46
Miscellaneous	
Foosh Energy Mints, 1 piece	100
Hershey's Special Dark Chocolate Bar, 1.45 ounces	18
Hershey's Chocolate Bar, 1.55 ounces	9
Hershey's Kisses, 9 pieces	9
Hot cocoa or chocolate milk, homemade, 8 ounces	5

Vitamins

Carbohydrates, protein, and fat supply fuel for cells, but these nutrients would be out of a job if it weren't for the vitamins that help the energy producers to function.

Vitamin A

Vitamin A is best known for its role in promoting peak vision, but it does much more than that. Vitamin A makes possible the growth and good health of cells and tissues throughout the body.

Vitamin A is actually a group of compounds that are important to reproduction, vision, and immunity. For a child developing in utero, vitamin A is necessary for cell division and for cell differentiation, which occurs during the first trimester, when the body decides which cells will become part of your baby's brain, muscle, bones, blood, and all other tissues.

Vitamin A comes in two forms. Retinol, which is ready-to-use vitamin A, is found largely in animal foods, such as liver and fortified milk, and in dietary supplements. Beta-carotene, alpha-carotene, and beta-cryptoxanthin are carotenoids (plant compounds) that the body is capable of converting to vitamin A. Brightly colored fruits and vegetables, including cantaloupe, sweet potatoes, and broccoli, offer carotenoids. Dietary supplements also contain carotenoids.

Although many Americans could use more carotenoids in their diet, studies suggest that few people are deficient in total vitamin A. However, you can have too much of a good thing. Excessive amounts of preformed (retinol) vitamin A, typically from supplements or acne medications, during early pregnancy can lead to birth defects.

In addition, studies suggest that excessive vitamin A intake hurts your bones. In a study published in the *Journal of the American Medical Association*, Harvard researchers found that women who consumed the most vitamin A as retinol from foods and supplements—more than three times the recommended amount—ran a significantly higher risk of hip fracture than those who ate close to the suggested amount. There is no evidence of a link between beta-carotene intake, especially from fruits and vegetables, and increased risk of osteoporosis, however.

DAILY NEEDS   The requirements for vitamin A are listed in micrograms (mcg) of retinol activity equivalents (RAE) to account for the different biological activities of retinol and for the carotenoids that become vitamin A in the body. Food and dietary supplement labels list vitamin A in international units (IU), but it's easy enough to do the conversion: 1 RAE equals 3.3 IU. It's not necessary to calculate the vitamin A you get from foods, but it is important to limit excessive amounts from supplements. Here's what you need every day:

- Nonpregnant (fourteen to fifty years old all ages): 700 mcg (2,310 IU)
- Pregnant: fourteen to eighteen years old, 750 mcg (2,475 IU); nineteen to fifty years old, 770 mcg (2,541 IU)
- Nursing: fourteen to eighteen years old, 1,200 mcg (3,960 IU); nineteen to fifty years old, 1,300 mcg (4,290 IU)

Do not consume more than 3,000 mcg (10,000 IU) of vitamin A at any time during your childbearing years. Taking in 10,000 IU or more a day has been associated with birth defects.

BEST FOOD SOURCES

Food	Vitamin A (mcg)
Sweet potato, ½ cup, baked	961
Carrot, ½ cup, chopped, raw	538
Spinach, ½ cup, cooked	472
Cantaloupe (a quarter of a whole cantaloupe)	467
Fortified breakfast cereals, 1 serving	150–230
Fortified milk, 2% reduced-fat, 8 ounces	134
Egg, 1 large, cooked any way	91

Vitamin D

Calcium might generate the most buzz for building strong bones, but it is nearly useless without vitamin D. Vitamin D oversees the absorption of calcium from food and supplements. Vitamin D also directs the movement of calcium in and out of bones, bolstering skeletal strength and allowing a healthy concentration of calcium in your bloodstream that promotes a regular heartbeat and normal muscle movement.

As nutrients go, vitamin D is a rarity. It's one of just two vitamins your body makes on its own. Exposure to strong sunshine triggers vitamin D production in the skin. The liver, kidneys, and cells in several other parts of the body convert vitamin D to its most potent form called cholecalciferol (vitamin D_3). Extra vitamin D is stored in your body fat for future use.

In theory, you can make all the vitamin D you need. In reality, many women do not. Living at latitudes above 40° North (about where Boston is located), where there's relatively weak sunshine for about half a year, plays a role in vitamin D deficiency. So does slathering on sunscreen that has a sun protection factor (SPF) of 8 or above, because that blocks the ultraviolet B rays that generate vitamin D. Women of color who live in northern climates may be at particular risk for low vitamin D levels because darker skin contains more melanin. Melanin provides color, but it also blocks the production of vitamin D. In addition, few foods provide vitamin D.

Vitamin D and Mothers-to-Be

It's a good idea to get into the habit of maintaining beneficial levels of vitamin D to help yourself and your future child. Studies done with female animals suggest that vitamin D plays a role in fertility. Other studies, including some conducted by Harvard researchers, have shown that vitamin D helps to fend off multiple sclerosis. Research also links adequate vitamin D levels in the blood to a lower risk of breast and ovarian cancer as well as a stronger immune system.

Once you're pregnant, vitamin D works in concert with calcium to promote the mineral's absorption from food and the deposition of it into your child's bones as well as yours. Women with higher vitamin D levels in their blood are at lower risk for preeclampsia, a condition of pregnancy that includes dangerously high blood pressure. Preeclampsia can slow a baby's growth in the womb, cause preterm delivery, and, if it becomes serious, result in death for you and your infant (see chapter 7 for more on preeclampsia, diet, and lifestyle).

Your getting the right amount of vitamin D can even help your child to avoid asthma. Two recent studies have linked higher vitamin D intake by the mother during pregnancy with a lower risk of recurrent wheeze or wheeze symptoms in the child's early years. In both studies, it didn't matter whether the mother's dietary vitamin D came from supplements or from foods.

DAILY NEEDS   Whether you're pregnant or not or you're nursing a child, you need at least 200 IU of vitamin D every day from age fourteen on. Don't worry that the 400 IU found in multivitamins and prenatal nutrition supplements might be excessive; according to the Institute of Medicine, 400 IU is perfectly safe every day. Limit vitamin D intake to the suggested upper limit of 2,000 IU per day, however.

Vitamin D: Meet Your Needs

Don't rely on your prenatal vitamin alone to fill vitamin D needs; food and sunshine count, too. A recent study in the *Journal of Nutrition* found low blood levels of vitamin D in pregnant women living in Pittsburgh, even though more than 90 percent of them took prenatal vitamin pills. Eight out of ten African American women and half of

WORDS OF
Motherly Wisdom

"To get the vitamin D
and calcium I needed, I
made chocolate milk in
a water bottle. Shaking
the milk instead of
stirring made it taste
like a milkshake!"
—*Robin*

the pregnant white women in the study
were deficient in vitamin D. The authors
concluded that higher doses of dietary
vitamin D are necessary to prevent the
low levels found in women living in the
northern regions of the United States,
about 40° North latitude and above.
Dark-skinned people in particular should
consider vitamin D supplements to meet
their needs. That's because the melanin
in darker skin acts as a natural sunscreen,
limiting the body's ability to produce
vitamin D.

BEST FOOD SOURCES   Few foods naturally supply vitamin D. Certain
fortified foods, including milk, yogurt, and 100% orange juice,
help to satisfy your need for this vital vitamin.

Food	Vitamin D (IU)
Salmon, 3½ ounces, cooked	360
Tuna, light, canned, drained, 3 ounces	200
Milk, all types, 8 ounces	100
Orange juice, fortified, 8 ounces	100
Yogurt, fortified, 6 to 8 ounces	80–100
Cereal, ready-to-eat, fortified, ¾ to 1 cup	40–60
Egg, 1 large, whole, cooked any way	20
Mushrooms, ½ cup, cooked	11

Vitamin E

The body's cells are under constant attack from free radicals, which are
unstable forms of oxygen that roam the body looking to make trouble. Free
radicals are by-products of normal, everyday metabolism, but they can
be lethal to cells by destroying the important fats in cell membranes.

Oxidative stress is the term that experts use to describe the havoc wreaked by free radicals. You can't escape free radicals, but you can limit their production by avoiding (as much as possible) smog and other air pollutants, cigarette smoking, secondhand smoke, and prolonged exposure to sunlight (ultraviolet rays).

As part of a healthy diet, vitamin E is one of the body's best weapons against daily oxidative stress. By donating part of itself to a free radical, vitamin E turns an unruly, hostile compound into a harmless substance, so the free radical is rendered incapable of destruction.

Vitamin E is garnering attention for another kind of defense: its ability to fend off oxidative damage to LDL cholesterol. It might seem strange to want to protect the "bad" cholesterol that clogs arteries, but when LDL cholesterol is oxidized by free radicals, it becomes stickier and more likely to clog arteries, boosting the risk of heart disease and stroke.

Vitamin E can also prevent blood cells from sticking to one another and to the blood vessels in which they travel, helping to promote clear and flexible blood vessels that allow the passage of oxygen-rich blood to your heart and, when you're pregnant, to the placenta, too.

Vitamin E is a fat-soluble vitamin, so it's mostly found in higher-fat foods, such as vegetable oils, margarine spreads, nuts, and seeds.

There are eight forms of vitamin E in foods, but one, alpha-tocopherol, is considered superior. Though important to your health, the other seven forms of vitamin E cannot meet the body's vitamin E needs. In fact, alpha-tocopherol is so potent that the recommended dietary allowance for vitamin E is based on the body's requirement for alpha-tocopherol. Even the synthetic form of alpha-tocopherol, which is found in fortified foods and supplements, is only half as effective in the body as the naturally occurring kind.

DAILY NEEDS

- Nonpregnant: all ages, 15 mg of alpha-tocopherol
- Pregnant: all ages, 15 mg of alpha-tocopherol
- Nursing: all ages, 19 mg of alpha-tocopherol
- Pregnant or nursing: limit intake of alpha-tocopherol to 800 mg if fourteen to eighteen years old and to 1,000 mg if nineteen to fifty years old

BEST FOOD SOURCES

Food	Vitamin E (as alpha-tocopherol, in mg)
Almond butter, 2 tablespoons	8
Almonds, raw or roasted, 1 ounce	7
Sunflower seeds, roasted, 1 ounce	7
Sunflower oil, 1 tablespoon	6
Safflower oil, 1 tablespoon	5
Wheat germ, 2 tablespoons	4
Hazelnuts, roasted, 1 ounce	4
Spinach, cooked, 1 cup	4
Peanut butter, 2 tablespoons	3
Peanuts, roasted, 1 ounce	2
Avocado (a quarter of a whole avocado)	2
Olive oil, 1 tablespoon	2
Broccoli, cooked, 1 cup	2
Kiwi, 1 medium	1

Vitamin K

Vitamin K has something in common with vitamin D: both are made by the body. Beneficial bacteria that are camped out in your digestive tract produce vitamin K, which is essential for normal blood clotting. Vitamin K is also necessary for the growth, development, and maintenance of bones because of its participation in the production of a number of proteins that contribute to skeletal strength.

Although vitamin K deficiency is rare, some people are more prone to it than others, such as people with celiac disease or ulcerative colitis. Certain medications, including antibiotics (for example, penicillin, amoxicillin, and sulfamethizole) and antiseizure drugs, interfere with vitamin K production by decreasing the bacteria in the intestinal tract that make vitamin K. Taking high doses of aspirin can interfere with the vitamin K balance in your body; so, too, can mineral oil, cholestyramine (to control cholesterol), and quinine or quinidine. Check with your doctor or pharmacist to determine your risk of vitamin K deficiency, and work with a registered dietitian to get the vitamin K you need if you take vitamin K–depleting medications on a long-term basis.

DAILY NEEDS   Vitamin K requirements do not increase with pregnancy or nursing; fourteen- to eighteen-year-olds need 75 mcg daily, and older women need 90 mcg. Although there is no evidence for an upper-limit requirement for vitamin K intake, there's no need to take vitamin K in supplement form, either. Newborns need a boost of vitamin K, however. The American Academy of Pediatrics recommends administering a single intramuscular injection of vitamin K_1 to all newborns to prevent vitamin K–deficiency bleeding, a potentially life-threatening condition.

BEST FOOD SOURCES

Food	Vitamin K (mcg)
Kale, cooked, 1 cup	1,146
Spinach, cooked, 1 cup	889
Brussels sprouts, 1 cup, cooked	229
Broccoli, 1 cup, cooked	220
Spinach, 1 cup, raw	145
Broccoli, 1 cup, raw	89
Asparagus, cooked, 8 spears	60
Lettuce, romaine, 1 cup	58
Peas, 1 cup, cooked	36
Soybeans, cooked, 1 cup	33
Kiwi, 1 medium	31
Blueberries, 1 cup	29

B Vitamins

B vitamins, such as B_2 (riboflavin), B_6, and B_{12}, perform similar functions. In general, they are vital to helping your body to derive energy from food, but each has a unique job, too. For example, vitamin B_{12} is useful for building robust blood cells; folate helps prevent birth defects; and pantothenic acid (vitamin B_5) is necessary for hormone production. B vitamins are found in abundance in a variety of foods, including fortified grains.

Vitamin B_1 (Thiamin)

Thiamin is notable for its role in promoting a normal nervous system and normal heart function.

DAILY NEEDS

- Nonpregnant: fourteen to eighteen years old, 1.0 mg; nineteen to fifty years old, 1.1 mg

- Pregnant: all ages, 1.4 mg
- Nursing: all ages, 1.5 mg

BEST FOOD SOURCES

Food	Thiamin (mg)
Pork tenderloin, 3 ounces, cooked	0.8
Pecans, 1 ounce, roasted or raw	0.2
Lentils, cooked, ½ cup	0.2
Long-grain white rice, enriched, cooked, ½ cup	0.2
Whole wheat bread, 1 slice (equal to 1 ounce)	0.1

Vitamin B_2 (Riboflavin)

Riboflavin is necessary for energy production. It also assists the body in using the protein that's in the food you eat.

DAILY NEEDS

- Nonpregnant: fourteen to eighteen years old, 1.0 mg; nineteen to fifty years old, 1.3 mg
- Pregnant: all ages, 1.4 mg
- Nursing: all ages, 1.6 mg

BEST FOOD SOURCES

Food	Riboflavin (mg)
Raisin Bran cereal, 1 cup	1.7
Yogurt, plain, 1 cup	0.5
Mushrooms, 1 cup, cooked	0.5
Milk, 1% low-fat, 1 cup	0.5
Cottage cheese, low-fat, 1 cup	0.4

Niacin (Vitamin B_3)

Niacin is needed for energy metabolism and for the proper growth and development of cells and tissues, particularly in the skin, nerve system, and digestive tract.

DAILY NEEDS

- Nonpregnant: all ages, 14 mg
- Pregnant: all ages, 18 mg
- Nursing: all ages, 17 mg

Food	Niacin (mg)
Chicken, skinless, breast meat, 3 ounces, cooked	12
Tuna, light, canned, drained, 3 ounces	11
Salmon, 3 ounces, cooked	9
Beef, 95% lean, 3 ounces, cooked	5
Peanuts, 1 ounce, dry roasted	4
Lentils, cooked, ½ cup	1

Pantothenic Acid (Vitamin B_5)

Pantothenic acid is part of an enzyme that generates energy from food, thereby contributing to sustaining life and supporting growth. This same enzyme helps the body to make several important compounds including neurotransmitters, which foster communication among brain cells, hormones, cholesterol, and fat.

DAILY NEEDS

- Nonpregnant: all ages, 5 mg
- Pregnant: all ages, 6 mg
- Nursing, all ages, 7 mg

BEST FOOD SOURCES

Food	Pantothenic Acid (mg)
Yogurt, plain, low-fat, 8 ounces	1
Chicken, white meat, 3 ounces, cooked	1
Sweet potato, ½ cup, baked	1
Egg, 1 large, hard-cooked	0.7
Mushrooms, ½ cup, raw, chopped	0.7

Vitamin B_6

Vitamin B_6 aids in protein production for new cells, bolsters the immune system, and participates in red blood cell formation. Although a vitamin B_6 deficiency is unlikely, it can cause a type of anemia. In large doses vitamin B_6 can alleviate morning sickness, but talk to your doctor before taking 25 to 50 mg a day to help you feel better.

DAILY NEEDS

- Nonpregnant: fourteen to eighteen years old, 1.2 mg; nineteen to fifty years old, 1.3 mg

- Pregnant: all ages, 1.9 mg
- Nursing: all ages, 2.0 mg

BEST FOOD SOURCES

Food	Vitamin B_6 (mg)
Product 19 cereal, 1 cup	2.0
Garbanzo beans, canned, drained, 1 cup	1.1
Potato, 1 medium, baked, with skin	0.6
Top sirloin, 3 ounces, cooked	0.6
Chicken breast, skinless, 3 ounces, cooked	0.5
Pork tenderloin, 3 ounces, cooked	0.4
Halibut, 3 ounces, cooked	0.3

Vitamin B_{12}

Vitamin B_{12} assists in red blood cell production and helps the body to use fat and carbohydrates for energy. Women who eat very small amounts of animal products or who avoid them altogether can become deficient in vitamin B_{12} unless they take supplements, eat fortified foods, or both.

DAILY NEEDS

- Nonpregnant: all ages, 2.4 mcg
- Pregnant: all ages, 2.6 mcg
- Nursing: all ages, 2.8 mcg

BEST FOOD SOURCES

Food	Vitamin B_{12} (mcg)
Salmon, 3 ounces, cooked	5
Rainbow trout, 3 ounces, cooked	4
Tuna, light, canned, drained, 3 ounces	3
Beef, 3 ounces, cooked	2
Wheat Chex cereal, 1 cup	1

Folate: The B-Vitamin Superstar

Folate is a B vitamin that is found naturally in foods. Folic acid is its synthetic counterpart and is added to enriched grains and dietary supplements. Folate and folic acid are vital for producing new and healthy red blood cells, which are necessary for a developing baby and a healthy mother. Folic acid is best known for preventing neural tube defects

(NTDs), including spina bifida, the most common type. Spina bifida is the incomplete closure of the neural tube, which becomes your baby's spinal column and brain.

The neural tube develops within the first twenty-eight days of pregnancy—often before a woman even suspects that she's pregnant. The U.S. Public Health Service says that if all women of childbearing age without a history of an NTD-affected pregnancy consumed 400 mcg of folic acid daily—before and during early pregnancy—it would reduce by at least 70 percent the number of pregnancies affected by NTDs. There is also evidence that taking 400 mcg of folic acid daily will protect your baby from certain heart abnormalities, cleft lip, and cleft palate.

Folate's wonders don't stop with heading off birth defects early in pregnancy. Adequate levels of folate in the bloodstream are linked to adequate growth during pregnancy as well as lower risks of the following: anemia in the mother, miscarriage, preterm delivery, and low birth weight.

Women in their childbearing years (ages fourteen to fifty) who are capable of becoming pregnant should consume 400 mcg of folic acid daily from vitamin supplements, from foods fortified with folic acid, or from a combination of the two, *in addition to* the naturally occurring folate that they will get from foods such as legumes, 100% orange juice, and strawberries.

According to the Institute of Medicine, the body absorbs about 50 percent of the folate that naturally occurs in foods such as orange juice. In contrast, the body absorbs approximately 85 percent of the folic acid in fortified foods and 100 percent of the folic acid in a vitamin supplement that is taken on an empty stomach.

How Much Folic Acid per Serving?

When you are searching for foods rich in folic acid, what should you look for on the label? Since nearly all of the folate in a processed product—such as cereal, rice, bread, and pasta—is in the form of folic acid, it's easy to determine how much of that food meets your daily need of 400 mcg. For example, if one serving is defined as one cup, and one cup contains 50 percent of the Daily Value for folic acid (that is, 200 mcg), you have met half of your daily quota for folic acid as a woman who is not pregnant.

DAILY NEEDS   Women with diabetes, epilepsy, or obesity are at an increased risk of having a baby with an NTD and need larger doses of folic acid. Women who take trimethorpim, triamterene, carbamazepine, phenytoin, phenobarbital, and primidone are at risk of folate deficiency. Speak with your health-care provider before pregnancy about the right folic acid dose for you. Don't consume more than 1,000 mcg a day unless you are advised to do so by a licensed medical professional.

- Nonpregnant: all ages, 400 mcg
- Pregnant: all ages, 600 mcg
- Nursing: all ages, 500 mcg

BEST FOOD SOURCES

Food	Folate (mcg)
Whole Grain Total cereal, ¾ cup	807*
Wheat Chex cereal, 1 cup	404*
Spinach, cooked, 1 cup	263
White rice, enriched, cooked, 1 cup	195*
Lentils, cooked, ½ cup	179
Spaghetti, enriched, cooked, 1 cup	172*
Broccoli, 1 cup, cooked	168
Orange juice, 8 ounces	110
White beans, canned, drained, ½ cup	85
Strawberries, sliced, 1 cup	40
Bread, enriched, 2 slices	34*

*Contains folic acid, the synthetic form of folate that is added to grains and dietary supplements.

Choline

Choline is a nutrient that is essential for the normal functioning of all cells, especially those in the brain, the liver, and the central nervous system. Choline works in tandem with folic acid to promote proper nervous system development during pregnancy.

Choline can help to protect your baby from NTDs. A recent *American Journal of Epidemiology* study of a group of women found that those who consumed the most choline had a 72 percent lower risk of an NTD-affected pregnancy than the women with the lowest choline intakes.

Animal studies show that choline is critical for the development of the hippocampus, the brain's memory center. The hippocampus is one of the only areas in the brain that continues to produce nerve cells throughout life. During pregnancy, the baby's organ growth, particularly the growth of the brain, happens at lightning speed, and the mother's diet must supply the choline that the developing child requires.

Nevertheless, many women enter pregnancy with a choline deficiency. That's the conclusion of a study from Iowa State University, which determined that less than 90 percent of women and pregnant women get the amount of dietary choline recommended by the Institute of Medicine. Vegans and women following very low fat diets are at particular risk for inadequate choline intake.

Choline is widely available in the food supply, but certain foods are particularly concentrated in it: eggs, liver, pork, and beef. For example, two eggs supply more than half the choline you need daily before, during, and after pregnancy. Don't rely on multivitamin pills or prenatal supplements for choline. Most dietary supplements supply little or no choline. Be sure to satisfy your choline quota with a balanced eating plan that includes choline-rich foods every day.

DAILY NEEDS

- Nonpregnant: all ages, 425 mg
- Pregnant: all ages, 450 mg
- Nursing: all ages, 550 mg
- Do not consume more than 3,500 mg of choline daily.

BEST FOOD SOURCES

Food	Choline (mg)
Egg, 1 large*, cooked any way	125
Cod, Atlantic, 3 ounces, cooked	84
Ground beef, 3 ounces, cooked	83
Pork tenderloin, 3 ounces, cooked	76
Shrimp, 3 ounces, cooked	69
Salmon, 3 ounces, cooked	65
Chicken, 3 ounces, cooked	65
Broccoli or cauliflower, 1¼ cups, cooked	40
Wheat germ, 2 tablespoons	21

*All of the choline is found in the yolk.

Vitamin C

Vitamin C is best known for its role in building and maintaining a robust immune system that fights infection and helps to ward off cancer. However, vitamin C does much more. It bolsters bones, teeth, and connective tissue; keeps blood vessels strong and resilient; and promotes healthy red blood cells. Vitamin C also improves the absorption of iron from plant foods and iron-fortified grains, such as bread and pasta.

DAILY NEEDS   Do not consume more than 1,800 mg a day of vitamin C if you are fourteen to eighteen years old and are pregnant or nursing, and no more than 2,000 mg a day if you are nineteen or older and are pregnant or nursing.

- Nonpregnant: all ages, 75 mg
- Pregnant: fourteen to eighteen years old, 80 mg; nineteen to fifty years old, 85 mg
- Nursing: fourteen to eighteen years old, 115 mg; nineteen to fifty years old, 120 mg

BEST FOOD SOURCES

Food	Vitamin C (mg)
Red bell pepper, raw, chopped, 1 cup	283
Orange juice, 8 ounces	124
Strawberries, sliced, 1 cup	106
Grapefruit juice, 8 ounces	94
Broccoli, 1 cup, cooked	74
Orange, 1 medium	70
Tomato, 1 medium	32

Minerals

Minerals are part of every process that supports life—in your body and in your baby's body. For example, minerals are involved in the normal functioning of the muscles and the nervous system and in bolstering the immune system. Minerals also provide structural support, as part of the bones, teeth, and red blood cells. Your body doesn't make minerals, so you need to get them from food or from dietary supplements.

Iron

Iron is vital to the production of hemoglobin, the part of the red blood cells that ferries oxygen to the cells in your body and your child's body. That's important, given the rapid cell proliferation during pregnancy. Iron also plays a role in building a robust immune system and in energy production. Finally, iron is integral to the development of a child's brain and nervous system.

Given the surge in red blood cell production during pregnancy, it's easy to understand why pregnancy dramatically increases iron needs. Heading into pregnancy with adequate iron stores helps to prevent iron-deficiency anemia, the most common nutritional deficit in the world, during pregnancy. Stored iron can be mobilized when dietary intake is inadequate, but when iron levels are low, the red blood cells take priority at the expense of the brain and all of the other tissues that need iron.

The iron in food, except in eggs, is one of two types: heme or nonheme iron. (Egg iron is about half of each type.) Heme iron is the predominant form in animal foods, such as red meat, seafood, and poultry. Nonheme iron is the only form in plant foods and in fortified products, such as bread, cereal, pasta, and rice. The body absorbs heme iron far better than it absorbs nonheme iron.

Here are some ways to improve iron uptake by the body, no matter what the type:

- Don't sip coffee or tea (even decaffeinated) with meals; it decreases nonheme iron absorption.
- Pair vitamin C and nonheme iron to significantly increase iron uptake by the body. For instance, combine the following: orange juice and iron-fortified breakfast cereal; strawberries and a sandwich made with fortified bread; iron-enriched pasta and tomato

---

Iron On Board

Most babies are born with a six-month supply of iron, but some have less at birth. Preterm infants, babies who did not grow properly in the womb, and children born to women with diabetes are prone to iron deficiency because they have less than optimal iron reserves at birth.

---

sauce; and burgers (ground turkey or beef) on iron-enriched rolls and a slice of tomato.

- Take your prenatal pill or iron supplements on an empty stomach, if possible.

DAILY NEEDS

- Nonpregnant: all ages, 8 mg
- Pregnant: all ages, 27 mg
- Nursing (if periods have resumed): all ages, 8 mg
- Nursing (if periods have not resumed): all ages, 9 mg

BEST FOOD SOURCES

Food	Iron (mg)
Whole Grain Total cereal, ¾ cup	22*
Cheerios, 1 cup	10*
Rice, enriched, cooked, 1 cup	8*
Oatmeal, instant, 1 packet	8*
Spinach, cooked, 1 cup	6
Soybeans, cooked, ½ cup	5
White beans, canned, drained, ½ cup	4
Beef, 3 ounces, cooked	3
Lamb, 3 ounces, cooked	2
Chicken breast, skinless, 3 ounces, cooked	1

*Contains added nonhence iron.

Zinc

Zinc is an all-around nutrient but is little known for its many vital functions. For example, zinc helps to produce DNA, the blueprint for every budding cell in your body and your baby's body. It is also involved in energy production and is necessary for brain development. Zinc is part of insulin, the hormone that regulates blood glucose levels, and it contributes to a healthy immune system and wound healing. These are just some of the ways that zinc promotes good health.

Zinc is particularly abundant in animal foods, including meat and certain seafood. Many breakfast cereals are fortified with zinc. Because zinc is primarily found in the germ and bran portions of grains, milling—a process used to make refined grains, which are then used to make white bread and crackers—removes up to 80 percent of the zinc from these grains.

Vegetarians and vegans may require as much as 50 percent more zinc than meat eaters because of certain elements in food that impair zinc uptake by the body. If you avoid animal products or eat very few on a regular basis, be sure to choose whole-grain foods (like brown rice or whole-wheat bread) and fortified grains, as part of a balanced diet, and take a multivitamin pill with 100 percent of the Daily Value for zinc before, during, and after pregnancy.

DAILY NEEDS

- Nonpregnant: all ages, 8 mg
- Pregnant: fourteen to eighteen years old, 12 mg; nineteen to fifty years old, 11 mg
- Nursing: fourteen to eighteen years old, 13 mg; nineteen to fifty years old, 12 mg
- Do not consume more than 40 mg of zinc a day from supplements.

BEST FOOD SOURCES

Food	Zinc (mg)
Oysters, 3 ounces, cooked	76
Whole Grain Total cereal, ¾ cup	17
Beef, 3 ounces, cooked	9
Lamb, 3 ounces, cooked	5
Crab, 3 ounces, cooked	5
Turkey, skinless, dark meat, 3 ounces, cooked	4
Pork, 3 ounces, cooked	4
White beans, canned, drained, ½ cup	2
Yogurt, plain, fat-free, 1 cup	2
Wheat germ, 2 tablespoons	2

Calcium

Calcium is the most ubiquitous of elements in the human body. It plays a central part in the function of nearly every cell, in addition to its best-known role of building and maintaining strong bones and teeth. Although your skeleton harbors nearly all of the calcium in your body, about 1 percent is in the blood and the tissues, perpetuating life by promoting normal muscle contraction, nerve transmission, and a regular heartbeat. When you don't get enough calcium in your diet, the body withdraws the mineral from your bones to keep blood calcium concentration within a healthy range.

During pregnancy, a woman's body becomes superefficient at absorbing calcium, which is why calcium quotas do not change. However, most women enter pregnancy deficient in calcium. In fact, only a small percentage of women in their childbearing years consume the calcium they need every day. Multivitamin pills and prescription prenatal supplements won't meet your calcium needs. You must get the calcium you require from foods and from calcium supplements, if necessary.

Dairy foods are dense in calcium. Women who completely avoid dairy foods or eat them sparingly might not get the calcium they require. To make matters worse, calcium absorption is often less efficient in a diet based solely on plant foods. High levels of oxalic and phytic acids (found in grains, legumes, nuts, and seeds) are known to interfere with calcium absorption. That's not to say that these foods are unhealthy; just the opposite. However, vegans, and other people who don't consume the recommended three servings of dairy foods daily, must get the calcium they need from fortified plant foods, such as 100% orange juice and soy beverages, from dietary supplements, or from a mixture of foods and supplements.

> WORDS OF
> *Motherly Wisdom*
>
> "As a vegan, I don't drink milk or eat dairy products, but I do make sure I get the calcium I need from a variety of calcium-added foods and foods that naturally contain calcium, too."
> —Dina

DAILY NEEDS

- Nonpregnant: fourteen to eighteen years old, 1,300 mg; nineteen to fifty years old, 1,000 mg
- Pregnant: fourteen to eighteen years old, 1,300 mg; nineteen to fifty years old, 1,000 mg
- Nursing: fourteen to eighteen years old, 1,300 mg; nineteen to fifty years old, 1,000 mg
- Do not consume more than 2,500 mg of calcium on a daily basis.

BEST FOOD SOURCES   Use the following list to determine the amount of calcium you get every day. If you don't typically get enough calcium from foods, see "The Best Calcium Supplements" sidebar below for which supplements to take.

Food	Calcium (mg)
Yogurt, plain, low-fat, 1 cup	415
Yogurt, fruit-flavored, low-fat, 1 cup	345
Milk, plain or flavored, 1 cup	300
Milk, lactose-free, 1 cup	300
Orange juice, calcium-added, 8 ounces	300
Cheddar cheese, 1 ounce	204
Tofu, firm, prepared with calcium sulfate and magnesium chloride, a quarter of a block	163
Cottage cheese, low-fat, 1 cup	138
Ice cream, vanilla, 1 cup	168
Broccoli, 1 cup, cooked	94

The Best Calcium Supplements

It's not only how much calcium you take, it's the quality that matters, too. Pills that contain calcium carbonate (such as Tums) and calcium citrate are highly favorable because they are the most readily absorbed forms. Calcium citrate malate (CCM) is a form of calcium that is used to fortify certain juices. Choose juices with CCM; it's absorbed well by the body. Don't take more than 500 mg of supplemental calcium at a time; separating calcium doses promotes peak absorption.

Magnesium

Magnesium is needed by every cell in your body and your baby's body. It helps to regulate muscle and nerve function, keeps the heart rhythm steady, and bolsters immunity. It's also important for promoting normal blood pressure and boosting bone strength. Magnesium is involved in energy metabolism and protein production, too.

DAILY NEEDS   There is no recommended upper limit for magnesium from food. However, do not consume more than 350 mg of magnesium

---

Disguising Dairy

What if you don't like dairy? Maybe you avoid dairy because of lactose intolerance. Women with lactose intolerance should seek out lactose-free milk and other lactose-reduced dairy foods. Try lactase products; they break down the lactose in foods for you. Work in more dairy with these easy tips:

- Prepare pudding with fat-free milk.
- Stir ricotta cheese or pureed cottage cheese into warm or cold pasta dishes.
- Make a fruit smoothie with yogurt or milk.
- Enjoy hot chocolate made with low-fat or fat-free milk.
- Prepare pancakes using yogurt (see chapter 8).
- Make mashed potatoes with evaporated milk instead of regular milk. Evaporated milk has twice the calcium.
- Prepare condensed soups with 1% low-fat or fat-free milk.
- Make oatmeal with milk in the microwave instead of water.

---

from dietary supplements or medications. Some laxatives, such as Milk of Magnesia, contain magnesium. Large doses of magnesium can cause diarrhea and abdominal cramping. Ask your doctor about alternatives when you're pregnant and nursing.

- Nonpregnant: fourteen to eighteen years old, 360 mg; nineteen to fifty years old, 310 mg
- Pregnant: fourteen to eighteen years old, 400 mg; nineteen to fifty years old, 350 mg
- Nursing: fourteen to eighteen years old, 360 mg; nineteen to fifty years old; 310 mg

BEST FOOD SOURCES

Food	Magnesium (mg)
Spinach, cooked, 1 cup	156
Artichoke hearts, 1 cup	101
Halibut, 3 ounces, cooked	91

Food	Magnesium (mg)
Brown rice, long-grain, cooked, 1 cup	84
Almonds, 1 ounce, roasted	78
Cashews, 1 ounce, roasted	77
Soybeans, cooked, ½ cup	74
Orange juice, 8 ounces	72
Potato, 1 medium, baked, with skin	57
Peanuts, 1 ounce, roasted	50
Whole-wheat bread, 2 slices	46
Baked beans, canned, ½ cup	43
Lentils, cooked, ½ cup	35
Milk, 8 ounces	34
Broccoli, 1 cup, cooked	33
Banana, 1 medium	32

Sodium

You might think of sodium as culpable for high blood pressure and bloating. That's true; sodium helps your body to hold on to fluid, which can cause swelling as well as elevated blood pressure. However, sodium is also beneficial. That's because your body, and your baby's body, is mostly water.

Maintaining a normal fluid balance is critical to a healthy blood pressure, no matter what your life stage. Even though sodium is often maligned, it is necessary for normal muscle contraction and nerve conduction. Sodium also transports nutrients into cells and carries waste products for removal from the body.

Sodium is a component of nearly every food, so you can't completely avoid it, but you can minimize its intake. Fresh foods are relatively low in sodium, whereas processed fare—such as fast foods, canned soups and vegetables, and frozen dinners—have the most. Most of the sodium we consume is found in processed and prepared foods; a mere 15 percent or so is actually from the salt shaker. Processed foods are rich in added salt (sodium chloride), but they

WORDS OF
Motherly Wisdom

"I never realized how much sodium was in the foods I ate on a daily basis until I started reading food labels. Now I go for lower-sodium versions whenever I can."
—Shana

often also contain sodium-laden additives such as monosodium gluta-mate (MSG), sodium citrate, and disodium phosphate.

DAILY NEEDS   Adults—pregnant, nursing, or not—should limit sodium intake to 2,300 mg a day, according to the Dietary Guidelines for Americans 2005. Check out the list below for sources of sodium in common foods.

BEST FOOD SOURCES

Food	Sodium (mg)
Salt, 1 teaspoon	2,300
Grilled chicken sandwich, fast-food	1,237
Soy sauce, 1 tablespoon	1,024
Cottage cheese, 1% low-fat, 1 cup	918
Pizza, frozen, 4 ounces	890
Soup, canned, 1 cup	700–1,200
Vegetable juice, canned, 8 ounces	653
Corn, canned, drained, 1 cup	571

Potassium

Potassium is essential for the body's growth and maintenance. It works with sodium to promote balance between the cells and the body's fluids. Potassium also plays an essential role in the response of the nerves to stimulation and in proper muscle contraction. Cellular enzymes need potassium to work properly, and muscles require potassium to store carbohydrates to use as energy. Potassium helps to shore up bones by counteracting calcium losses from the body caused by high-sodium diets.

All foods contain potassium, but fresh foods contain the most. Processing destroys potassium. Everyone needs 4,700 mg of potassium daily. That goes for pregnant and nursing women of all ages, too.

BEST FOOD SOURCES

Food	Potassium (mg)
Winter squash, cubed, 1 cup, cooked	896
Sweet potato, 1 medium, baked, with skin	694
Potato, 1 medium, baked, with skin	610
White beans, canned, drained, ½ cup	595
Yogurt, fat-free, 1 cup	579

Food	Potassium (mg)
100% orange juice, 8 ounces	496
Halibut, 3 ounces, cooked	490
Broccoli, 1 cup, cooked	457
Cantaloupe, cubed, 1 cup	431
Banana, 1 medium	422
Honeydew melon, cubed, 1 cup	388
Pork tenderloin, 3 ounces, cooked	383
Lentils, cooked, ½ cup	366
Black-eyed peas, cooked, ½ cup	345
Raisins, ¼ cup	250
Chicken breast, 3 ounces, cooked	218
Almonds, 1 ounce, roasted	211
Tuna, light, canned, drained, 3 ounces	201

Iodine

Iodine is a major component of the thyroid hormones that regulate a number of key biochemical reactions in the body, including protein production and metabolic rate. During pregnancy, thyroxine and other hormones are necessary for the myelination of the nervous system, a process that ensures speedy and correct communication among the nerve cells and in the brain. Inadequate iodine intake during pregnancy takes a toll on the baby's brain development and can lead to very serious effects, including mental retardation.

DAILY NEEDS

- Nonpregnant: all ages, 150 mcg
- Pregnant: all ages, 220 mcg
- Nursing: all ages, 290 mcg
- Limits of daily intake: nonpregnant, pregnant, and nursing, fourteen to eighteen years old, 900 mcg; nineteen to fifty years old, 1,100 mcg

BEST FOOD SOURCES   Iodized salt—table salt with iodine added—provides much of the iodine in the American diet. Seafood is naturally rich in iodine; cod, sea bass, haddock, and perch are all good sources. Kelp, a common sea vegetable, is also rich in iodine. Dairy products, and plants grown in iodine-rich soil, contain iodine, too. A quarter teaspoon of iodized table salt provides 95 mcg of iodine. A six-ounce portion of ocean fish provides 650 mcg of iodine. Most people are able to meet the daily recommendations by eating seafood, iodized salt, and plants grown in iodine-rich soil. When you buy salt, make sure it is labeled "iodized." Processed foods may also be rich in iodine if they contain iodized salt or additives such as calcium iodate or cuprous iodide. However, iodine content is not typically listed on food labels, so it's unclear how much iodine you're getting in a serving.

Phytonutrients: Neither Vitamins nor Minerals

Ellagic acid, phenethyl isothiocyanate, lutein, zeaxanthin, and sulforaphane—this sounds like a mess of chemicals you'd find in the most processed foods. However, these compounds, collectively known as *phytochemicals* or *phyto-nutrients*, are naturally occurring substances in plant foods. Phytonutrients are credited for having a multitude of health benefits, including reducing heart disease, boosting immunity, lowering the risk of certain cancers, and improving eyesight.

Many phytonutrients serve more than one purpose. Some provide pigments that brighten fruits and vegetables, including blueberries, watermelon, and cantaloupe. Others repel damage to their host plants from germs or strong sunlight. Still other phytonutrients, such as beta-carotene, serve as the raw material for vitamin A in the body. Beta-carotene also helps to thwart cell damage that could threaten your health and your child's development.

Nobody knows exactly how many beneficial substances lurk in plant foods, but it's probably more than ten thousand. The list seems to grow every week. Brightly colored fruits and vegetables, such as tomatoes, broccoli, oranges, spinach, carrots, and sweet potatoes are among the foods richest in phytonutrients. Whole grains are a good source of phytonutrients, too.

Now You Know

Now that you've read this chapter, you've learned a lot. You know that some fats are better than others, that you don't have to drink plain water to satisfy fluid needs, what the latest research says about caffeine limits before and during pregnancy, and much more. Don't worry if you don't recall everything you read; you know where to find the information.

The next chapter takes you another step in your quest to learn more about the best diet before, during, and after pregnancy. Chapter 3 discusses healthy eating plans that incorporate all the goodness of the nutrients you read about in this chapter. Chapter 3 also details MyPyramid, a balanced approach to a healthy eating plan that nearly all women, and their partners, can easily follow.

3

MyPyramid Plans: What to Eat Before, During, and After Pregnancy

Chapter 2 covered the nutrients that are considered critical to the good health of you and your baby. However, you don't eat nutrients, you eat food. That's why you need a guide for what foods and how much of them to include in a nutritious eating plan. This chapter helps you, and your partner, to build a balanced diet while adhering to a calorie level that's just right.

MyPyramid and Yours

You may have grown up with the Food Guide Pyramid, which was designed to help Americans to eat healthily. There's a new pyramid now: MyPyramid, which replaced the Food Guide Pyramid in 2005. MyPyramid provides an easy way to get the nutrients you need from each food group every day; it's for most healthy people ages two and older, including pregnant and nursing women.

MyPyramid supplies advice about how much to eat from each of the five foods groups (grains, vegetables, fruits, milk, and meat and beans) and from fats and oils. MyPyramid's dietary recommendations are based on the most current scientific evidence. In fact, MyPyramid follows the guidance given in the Dietary Guidelines for Americans 2005, which are published by the U.S. Department of Health and Human Services and the U.S. Department of Agriculture.

Balance, variety, and moderation rule the pyramid and its suggestions for healthy eating. MyPyramid includes physical activity recommendations, too. The best part of MyPyramid is that it gets personal. MyPyramid makes planning a balanced diet easier because it takes into account age, sex, and physical activity level, as well as whether you're pregnant or nursing.

When You Need More Help:
Ask a Registered Dietitian

MyPyramid serves as an excellent foundation for a healthy weight, but you may need more assistance with your eating plan because of a chronic condition, such as an eating disorder, diabetes, or high blood pressure. Perhaps you just want more information about building a better diet. In that case, consult a registered dietitian (RD). RDs have a minimum of a bachelor's degree from an accredited college or university, and they've also completed an accredited preprofessional experience program, such as a twelve-month internship at a hospital. Many RDs hold advanced degrees. RDs are trained to tailor an eating plan to your needs, accounting for your medical history, goals, and life stage. For a free referral to an RD in your area, go to www.eatright.org and click on "Find a Nutrition Professional" on the home page.

Determining Your Physical Activity Level

You already know what sex you are and your age. You need one more piece of information to take the first step to better eating: your physical activity level. Along with age and sex, physical activity determines daily calorie allowances.

Every move you make uses calories. However, you might give yourself more credit than you deserve for calorie burning. You're not alone—most people overestimate their physical activity. Doing so can backfire, because you might eat more than you should, based on your perceived activity. Overeating can result in weight gain and frustration when the pounds won't come off.

Surely any movement is better than nothing, but some movements are better than others. For example, it's more beneficial to stroll for thirty minutes a day than it is to get off the couch thirty times a night after dinner to change the television channel. Even so, getting up is better than using the remote control while lounging on the couch, because doing so uses energy.

Walking, biking, swimming, hiking, aerobics, and strength training are the best activities because they strengthen your heart, lower your blood pressure, and reduce risk for certain cancers. The Dietary Guidelines for Americans 2005 and MyPyramid stress a minimum of thirty minutes of physical activity each day for adults. We discuss the guidelines for exercise during pregnancy in chapter 4.

Use the following guidelines to determine your physical activity:

If you exercise . . .	Then you're . . .
Less than 30 minutes on most days	Sedentary
30 to 60 minutes on most days	Moderately active
60 to 90 minutes on most days	Active

Your Daily Calorie Needs Made Easy

Now that you've figured out your physical activity level, it's time to select a daily calorie quota. The calorie levels in the chart on page 74, from MyPyramid, serve as guidelines to promote weight maintenance in men and in women who are either not pregnant or are in their first trimester. Pick a calorie level based on your age, sex, and physical activity level; this will be the number of calories you should eat if you're not pregnant and you want to maintain your weight, or if you're less than thirteen weeks pregnant. If you are not pregnant and you'd like to shed some pounds prior to conceiving, see the MyPyramid Prepregnancy Plan (on page 74) for how to proceed. If you're pregnant and past the first trimester, or are nursing, read on for more information about your daily suggested calorie budget.

DAILY CALORIE NEEDS

Age	Calorie Level		
	Sedentary	Moderately Active	Active
Women			
14–18	1,800	2,000	2,400
19–25	2,000	2,200	2,400
26–30	1,800	2,000	2,400
31–50	1,800	2,000	2,200
Men			
16–18	2,400	2,800	3,200
19–20	2,600	2,800	3,000
21–35	2,400	2,800	3,000
36–40	2,400	2,600	2,800
41–55	2,200	2,400	2,800

The MyPyramid Prepregnancy Plan

Choosing a calorie level was pretty painless, right? You're not done yet, however. If you're not pregnant, you have a decision to make: lose weight, stay the same, or add some pounds. If you are more than thirteen weeks pregnant, skip to the MyPyramid Pregnancy Plan on page 76. If you're nursing, see the MyPyramid Postpregnancy Plan on page 77.

To know what to do about your weight, you will need to know your body mass index (BMI) first, if you don't already (see chapter 1). Knowing your BMI informs you about whether to lose weight, gain some pounds, or stay the same before getting pregnant.

As we discussed in chapter 1, starting pregnancy at a healthy weight is very important to your child's growth and development and to your health, too. Losing weight prior to pregnancy isn't just for women, however. Get your partner involved in gradually adopting a lifestyle that incorporates good nutrition and regular physical activity. Healthy habits benefit both of you by possibly decreasing fertility problems. Adopting a nutritious diet before your baby is born makes it easier to stay on track later, when life gets busier.

You may be eager to drop some pounds and get on with starting a family, but you must allow a reasonable amount of time to lose the weight.

Cutting calories, increasing physical activity, or both will help you to shed pounds. If you want to lose about two pounds a week, shave 500 calories from your daily calorie allowance, exercise more, or do both. A two-pound weekly weight loss (or less) is considered safest.

You will need to rely more on the slimming effects of physical activity than calorie reduction if your maintenance calorie needs are 1,800 or 2,000 a day. That's because you should not eat fewer than 1,600 calories daily. Undereating will speed up the weight loss, but it makes it very difficult for you to get the nutrients—including protein, iron, and folic acid—that are necessary to prime your body for pregnancy. Furthermore, it's hard to stick with lower-calorie eating regimens (under 1,600 calories a day). Instead of cheating yourself of good nutrition and eating satisfaction, use this time as an opportunity to build a better diet that benefits you and your future child.

If you become overwhelmed by thinking that weight loss means dietary deprivation that you cannot live with, consider this. Even small changes in calorie consumption can shrink your waistline with time. For example, cutting back by 100 calories every day (the equivalent of one ounce of potato chips or two small crème-filled cookies) and burning an extra 100 calories can produce a ten-pound weight loss in about six months.

Physical activity enhances weight-loss efforts, particularly when combined with a lower-calorie eating plan. Start exercising on a regular basis, if you don't do so already. Try to fit in a minimum of thirty minutes of moderate activity, like walking, on most days of the week. Women with medical conditions should speak with their health-care provider before starting an exercise program. Let your doctor know that you're embarking on a healthier eating and exercise regimen to get in better shape before you conceive.

To gain weight, add 250 to 500 calories a day to your calorie budget. Keep track of what you're taking in, and be sure it measures up to what your MyPyramid plan suggests. You could be satisfying your daily calorie quota but underestimating your physical activity, so you would need to eat more to put on the pounds. If you're not able to put on some weight, seek help from an RD.

> WORDS OF
> *Motherly Wisdom*
>
> "Having an eating plan to go by is definitely a plus, but you don't have to adhere to it 100 percent of the time to get good results."
> —*Sarah*

The MyPyramid Pregnancy Plan

Even when you're pregnant, you might not need to eat more. During the first trimester (the first thirteen weeks of pregnancy), continue to follow your MyPyramid Prepregnancy Plan. If you were trying to lose weight prior to conception, stop now. Add back the calories you cut from your diet.

Using MyPyramid as the blueprint for your prepregnancy eating plan makes it easy to figure out what to eat during pregnancy. Eating according to MyPyramid will help you to gain the right amount of weight while getting the nutrients you need to nourish yourself and your growing baby.

A full-term (forty-week) pregnancy requires tens of thousands of calories to fuel. Although you may feel hungrier at times and experience more food cravings during the first weeks of pregnancy, calorie needs won't increase until the end of the first trimester. That makes sense, given that after the initial thirteen weeks of pregnancy, your baby is only about as big as your thumb. The baby's size doesn't diminish the importance of your diet, however; rather, it intensifies it. That's because the need for many important nutrients, particularly folic acid, surge once you're pregnant, even though calorie requirements have not yet caught up.

A child begins growing in earnest at the start of the second trimester. Once you've passed the thirteenth week, your daily calorie budget increases by about 330 calories. In the third trimester, you need 450 more calories every day than you did in the first trimester or when you're not pregnant. Perhaps you envision spending your calorie windfall on brownie sundaes or a huge pile of nachos and cheese, but that's not a good idea on a regular basis. Adding calories isn't enough—you need to make them work for you and your baby. Make the most of extra food by including healthy choices the majority of the time. That doesn't mean you can't indulge occasionally, however.

Here are some ways to "spend" extra pregnancy calories. The following combinations contain about 330 calories:

- One cup of whole-grain cereal with eight ounces of 1% low-fat milk and a quarter cup of dried cranberries
- Eight ounces of vanilla low-fat yogurt mixed with one ounce of slivered almonds
- A medium pear with one and a half ounces of reduced-fat cheese and six whole-grain crackers

- A medium apple smeared with two tablespoons of peanut butter, almond butter, or sunflower seed butter, along with eight ounces of fat-free milk
- Two hard-cooked eggs and half a whole-grain bagel with one teaspoon of trans fat–free tub margarine and one teaspoon of jam

The following choices provide about 450 calories:

- A one-ounce bagel topped with half a cup of low-fat cottage cheese, along with eight ounces of low-sodium vegetable juice
- A nut butter and banana sandwich: two slices of whole-wheat bread, two tablespoons of peanut butter, almond butter, or sunflower seed butter, and half a large banana or two tablespoons of raisins
- Three ounces of roasted chicken, one medium baked sweet potato with two teaspoons of trans fat–free tub margarine, along with eight ounces of 1% low-fat chocolate milk
- Four ounces of cooked lean beef and two ounces of whole-grain bread
- A fruit smoothie made with one cup of 1% low-fat milk, one cup of fresh or frozen berries, and one teaspoon of sugar, along with a two-ounce bagel with two teaspoons of trans fat–free tub margarine

The MyPyramid Postpregnancy Plan

Once you've had the baby, you'd like to have your body back. That's a reasonable desire, but it won't happen instantly. For many women, regaining their figure is a slow and steady process that can take several months to a year. If you're not nursing, refer to the MyPyramid Prepregnancy Plan to get back on a healthy eating regimen.

> WORDS OF
> *Motherly Wisdom*
>
> "When I found out I was pregnant the first time, it was a bit of an eating free-for-all at first! But I managed to get on track and ate right the rest of my pregnancy."
> —Deb

Whether you're breast-feeding or not, don't begin restricting calories for at least six weeks after your delivery day. Your body needs time to recover, and you should not shortchange your diet in order to fit into your prepregnancy clothes. You need all the strength you can muster to care for a newborn.

During the first six months, nursing women require almost as many calories as during the second trimester: 330 calories a day more than prepregnancy needs. After six months, you need about 400 calories a day, or close to what you were eating during the third trimester. The actual calorie cost of producing milk to nourish a child is more than 330 or 400 calories, but the body mobilizes some of the fat stored during pregnancy for energy to make breast milk.

Putting It All Together: The MyPyramid Plans

It's not enough to know how many calories you need at each stage of life. In order to construct a balanced eating plan, you must keep in mind both the number and the size of the servings to select from each food group in MyPyramid. To find out how many servings are right for you, locate the calorie level you've selected from the table below.

NUMBER OF SERVINGS PER FOOD GROUP

Calorie Level	Food Groups					
	Grains	Vegetables	Fruits	Fats and Oils	Milk	Meat and Beans
1,600	5	2	1.5	5	3	5
1,800	6	2.5	1.5	5	3	5
2,000	6	2.5	2	6	3	5.5
2,200	7	3	2	6	3	6
2,400	8	3	2	7	3	6.5
2,600	9	3.5	2	8	3	6.5
2,800	10	3.5	2.5	8	3	7
3,000	10	4	2.5	10	3	7
3,200	10	4	2.5	11	3	7

The Five Food Groups

Most foods, including chocolate bars, snack chips, and foot-long hot dogs, fit into a balanced diet. Eating any food in the right portions is the key to controlling calories and to good nutrition. This section delves into each of the five food groups in MyPyramid, explaining why the foods are good for you and how much of each constitutes a serving.

The Grain Group

Grain foods—such as bread, rice, and pasta—are a major source of carbohydrates, the body's preferred source of energy. Grains contain several B vitamins that help your body to harness the energy from food and make it useful to you and your developing baby. Enriched and fortified grains supply additional nutrients, such as folic acid and iron.

When you are choosing from the grain group, pick foods (cereals, breads, pasta) that are rich in whole grains for at least half of the grain servings that your MyPyramid eating plan allows. Whole grains are typically higher in fiber, certain vitamins and minerals, and phytonutrients than their refined counterparts (found in such foods as white bread, pretzels, some brands of breakfast cereals, and cookies). A diet rich in whole grains has been linked to a lower risk of heart disease, cancer, and diabetes, and it is helpful with weight control.

A whole-grain product may be produced from any type of grain, including wheat, oats, corn, rice, and barley. Check the label to be sure the food is rich in unrefined grains. Ingredients are listed in descending order, so look for the word *whole* in front of the name of the grain as the primary ingredient. Foods made only with bran are not whole-grain products. When you are evaluating claims on food labels such as "made with whole grains," it's useful to know that the bare minimum for whole-grain consumption is 48 grams per day.

Health claims about whole grains are regulated by the Food and Drug Administration. A manufacturer may choose to include a health claim linking a diet rich in whole grains to a reduced risk of heart disease and certain types of cancer when the product contains all portions of the grain kernel and a minimum of 51 percent whole grain by weight. The product must also meet specified levels for fat, cholesterol, and sodium. See the list below for grain foods and their portion sizes.

Food	Portion Size
Bagel	1 ounce (e.g., 1 mini)
Biscuits	1 small (2" in diameter)
Bread	1 regular slice; 1 small slice French; or 4 snack-size slices
Bulgur	½ cup cooked
Cornbread	1 small piece (2½" × 1¼" × 1¼")

(continued)

Food	**Portion Size** (*continued*)
Crackers	5 whole-wheat crackers; 2 rye crisp breads; or 7 square or round crackers
English muffin	half of one muffin
Oatmeal	½ cup cooked; 1 instant packet; or 1 ounce dry (regular or quick cooking)
Pancakes	1 medium (4½" in diameter) or 2 small (3" in diameter)
Pasta (includes couscous)	½ cup cooked or 1 ounce dry
Popcorn	3 cups popped
Ready-to-eat cereal	1 cup flakes or rounds; or 1¼ cups puffed cereal
Rice	½ cup cooked or 1 ounce dry
Tortillas	1 small (6")

Preventing Portion Distortion

For weight control and a balanced diet, it's not always what you eat, but how much. When you're watching your weight, or when you're pregnant or nursing a child, portion size matters. Even when you're committed to eating healthily, it's sometimes impossible to weigh and measure foods. Portion control can literally be at your fingertips when you use this portable method to prevent portion distortion:

- Your fist is equal to about one cup of cooked rice, pasta, or other grains and veggies and fruits.
- Your palm (flat) is about the size of three ounces of red meat, fish, or poultry.
- Your palm (cupped) holds one ounce of nuts or raisins.
- A handful of chips, popcorn, or pretzels is about two ounces.
- Your thumb is about the size of one ounce of peanut butter or hard cheese.
- The tip of your thumb is about the size of one teaspoon of oil, mayonnaise, butter, or sugar.

The Vegetable Group

In MyPyramid, vegetables are not created equal. This does not mean that some are better for you than others, exactly. However, MyPyramid does recommend eating vegetables such as broccoli and carrots more often than cucumber and bean sprouts because the former (along with other deeply colored produce) tend to offer more vitamins, minerals, and fiber. The differences in nutrient content become apparent when you compare, for instance, the suggested portion for romaine lettuce (one cup) to its lighter cousin, iceberg lettuce (two cups). Even so, lighter-colored vegetables—such as onions, cauliflower, and white potatoes—supply a bevy of nutrients, too.

MyPyramid recommends a variety of produce, which is illustrated by the five categories within the vegetable group. By categorizing vegetables into subgroups and recommending how much to eat from each, MyPyramid encourages you to consume an array of nutrients, including carbohydrates, fiber, vitamins A and C, phytonutrients, and water.

You'll notice that dried beans (such as garbanzo beans, black beans, and kidney beans), peas, and tofu are included in MyPyramid's vegetable group. That's because they are indeed vegetables. These foods are also found in the pyramid's meat group because of their high protein levels, so eating beans, peas, and soy products double as servings from the meat group, too.

For the most part, pick the least-processed vegetable choices; they offer more fiber, vitamins, and minerals as well as less fat and fewer calories. For example, a medium baked potato supplies one and a half times the potassium of a medium order of fast-food french fries, with 223 fewer calories and 20 fewer grams of fat. See the following list for vegetable servings.

Food	Portion Size
Dark Green Vegetables	
Broccoli	1 cup chopped or florets or 3 spears, 5" long, raw or cooked
Collard greens, mustard greens, turnip greens, kale	1 cup cooked

(continued)

Food	**Portion Size** (*continued*)
Raw leafy greens (spinach, romaine, watercress, dark green leafy lettuce, endive, escarole)	2 cups

Orange Vegetables

Carrots	1 cup raw or cooked, sliced or chopped; or 2 medium whole 1 cup baby carrots (about 12)
Pumpkin	1 cup cooked and mashed
Sweet potato	1 large baked (2¼" or more in diameter) 1 cup cooked, sliced or mashed
Winter squash (acorn, butternut, hubbard)	1 cup cooked, cubed

Dried Beans and Peas

Dried beans and peas (black, garbanzo, kidney, pinto, soy, black-eyed, split, lentils)	1 cup cooked, whole or mashed
Tofu	1 cup (½" cubes), about 8 ounces

Starchy Vegetables

Corn, yellow or white	1 cup 1 large ear (8" to 9" long)
Green peas	1 cup
Potatoes	1 cup cooked, diced or mashed 1 medium, boiled or baked (2½" to 3" in diameter) French fries: 20 medium to long strips (2½" to 4" long)

Other

Bean sprouts*	1 cup cooked
Cabbage, green	1 cup raw or cooked, chopped or shredded

Cauliflower	1 cup raw or cooked, pieces or florets
Celery	1 cup raw or cooked, diced or sliced; or 2 large stalks (11" to 12" long)
Cucumbers	1 cup raw, sliced or chopped
Green or wax beans	1 cup cooked
Lettuce, iceberg	2 cups raw, shredded or chopped; or 1 head
Mushrooms	1 cup raw or cooked
Onions	1 cup raw or cooked, chopped
Tomatoes	1 large whole raw, 3" in diameter
	1 cup raw, canned, or cooked, chopped or sliced
Tomato or mixed vegetable juice**	1 cup
Summer squash or zucchini	1 cup cooked, sliced or diced

* Raw sprouts are hazardous to your health. Eat only cooked sprouts.

** Choose low-sodium varieties.

The Fruit Group

Understanding how to make choices from the offerings in the fruit group is far easier than navigating the vegetable group. Fruit also tends to be easier for some people to include in a balanced diet than a salad, broccoli, or brussels sprouts because it is sweet and appealing, tends to be portable, and involves minimal preparation.

Fruit offers carbohydrates, fiber, water, potassium, vitamins A and C, phytonutrients, and water. Including the suggested amount of fruit each day may make weight control easier because the fiber and water in fruit is filling. Consuming the right amount of fruit for your calorie budget reduces the temptation for higher-calorie treats, such as cookies and chips, and can lower your overall energy intake.

The majority of the fruit you eat should come from whole, unprocessed sources, but any fruit, including 100% fruit juice and dried fruit, counts toward your daily fruit quota. See the list on page 84 for fruit servings.

Food	Portion Size
Apple	½ large (3¼" in diameter); 1 small (2½" in diameter); or 1 cup raw or cooked, sliced or chopped
Applesauce	1 cup
Banana	1 large (8" to 9") or 1 cup sliced
Berries (excluding strawberries)	1 cup
Cantaloupe	1 cup diced or balls
Grapefruit	1 medium (4" in diameter) or 1 cup sections
Grapes	1 cup whole or cut up or 32 grapes
Mixed fruit (fruit cocktail)	1 cup
Orange	1 large (3" in diameter) or 1 cup sections
Orange, mandarin	1 cup canned, drained
Peach	1 large (2¾" in diameter); 1 cup raw, cooked, or canned and drained, sliced or diced; or 2 halves, canned
Pear	1 medium pear (2½ per pound) or 1 cup raw, cooked, or canned and drained, sliced or diced
Pineapple	1 cup raw, cooked, or canned and drained, chunks, sliced, or crushed
Strawberries	About 8 large berries or 1 cup fresh or frozen, whole, halved, or sliced
Watermelon	1 small wedge (1" thick) or 1 cup diced or balls
Dried fruit	¼ cup
100% fruit juice	1 cup

The Milk Group

"Drink your milk" is a favorite refrain of parents. You may have been admonished to drain your glass hundreds of times as a child, and for good reason. Milk is an excellent source of calcium and vitamin D. It also supplies protein, vitamin A, several B vitamins, and minerals. With the exception of providing vitamin D, most yogurt and cheese has a nutrient profile similar to milk's.

MyPyramid's milk group recommendations for adults is the easiest of all to remember: three cups of milk daily or the equivalent in dairy foods, no matter what calorie level you've chosen for yourself, whether you're pregnant or not, nursing, or a male. Reach for lower-fat dairy foods most of the time. Technically, you could choose three servings of ice cream every day to satisfy your milk group quota, but it would cost you far more in calories and saturated fat than choosing low-fat or fat-free milk, yogurt, and cheese, which keep calories and saturated fat to a minimum. See the following list for servings in the milk group.

Food	Portion Size
Milk	1 cup, any fat level, lactose-free included; or 1 half-pint container ½ cup evaporated milk
Yogurt	1 regular container (8 fluid ounces) or 1 cup
Cheese	1½ ounces hard cheese, such as American, cheddar, mozzarella, Swiss, and Parmesan ⅓ cup shredded cheese 2 ounces processed cheese ½ cup ricotta cheese 2 cups cottage cheese, any fat level
Milk-based desserts	1 cup pudding prepared with milk 1 cup frozen yogurt 1½ cups ice cream

The Meat and Beans Group

Meat and beans are grouped together because of the protein they provide. Protein explains the other members of this group, too, including eggs, seafood, mixed nuts, chicken, turkey, and tofu.

Protein may be the common denominator in the meat and beans group, but the idea is to select an array of foods from this category for a variety of nutrients, such as B vitamins, vitamin E, iron, zinc, magnesium, and fiber. Stick with lean cuts of beef, skinless poultry, eggs, nuts, dried peas and beans, and seafood to limit saturated fat intake and maximize nutrient density. See the list below for servings in the meat and beans group.

Food	Portion Size
Lean beef, cooked; ham, cooked; or pork, cooked	1 ounce
Chicken or turkey, no skin or bones, cooked	1 ounce
Sliced turkey sandwich meat	1 ounce
Fish or shellfish, cooked	1 ounce
Eggs	1 whole
Nuts	½ ounce (12 almonds, 24 pistachios, or 7 walnut halves)
Seeds	½ ounce
Almond butter	1 tablespoon
Peanut butter	1 tablespoon
Dried beans	¼ cup cooked
Dried peas	¼ cup cooked
Baked beans, refried beans	¼ cup
Lentil soup	½ cup
Split pea soup	½ cup
Bean soup	½ cup
Tofu	¼ cup (about 2 ounces)
Tempeh	1 ounce cooked
Soybeans, roasted	¼ cup
Falafel patty	1 (about 4 ounces)
Hummus	2 tablespoons

The Fats and Oils Group

Fats make food taste good, but they have more calories than carbohydrates and protein, so it's wise to limit your intake. Your MyPyramid eating plan actually provides an allowance for the oils found in fatty foods. The serving size in the fats and oils group is expressed as teaspoons of oil. For example, if you're allowed seven servings a day from the fats and oils group, then you should account for seven teaspoons of oil in your diet. The following list tells you the exact amount of oil found in certain oil-rich foods.

Food	Portion Size	Amount of Oil
Vegetable oil	1 tablespoon	3 teaspoons
Margarine, soft (trans fat–free)	1 tablespoon	2½ teaspoons
Mayonnaise	1 tablespoon	2½ teaspoons
Mayonnaise-based salad dressing	1 tablespoon	1 teaspoon
Italian dressing	2 tablespoons	2 teaspoons
Thousand Island dressing	2 tablespoons	2½ teaspoons
Olives, ripe, canned	4 large	½ teaspoon
Avocado	½ of a medium-size	3 teaspoons
Peanut butter	2 tablespoons	4 teaspoons
Peanuts, dry roasted	1 ounce	3 teaspoons
Cashews, dry roasted	1 ounce	3 teaspoons
Almonds, dry roasted	1 ounce	3 teaspoons
Hazelnuts	1 ounce	4 teaspoons
Sunflower seeds	1 ounce	3 teaspoons

Room for Fun

You're eating five servings of fruits and vegetables every day, and you're also achieving your quotas for low-fat dairy foods, lean protein sources, and whole grains. Is there any room for cookies, candy, and cake in MyPyramid's plan for healthy eating? You bet!

Each MyPyramid calorie level reserves about 10 to 15 percent of its energy as *discretionary calories*. These are calories that are left over after you have satisfied your nutrient needs by choosing the suggested number of lower-calorie foods from each of the food groups.

Think of discretionary calories as what you can spend on any food you like—as long as it's safe, that is, especially during pregnancy and lactation. For example, a 2,000-calorie eating plan allows for nearly 300 discretionary calories. You can spend them on extra bread or meat or on three crème-filled sandwich cookies and eight ounces of 1% low-fat milk. No questions asked!

Sample Meal Plans

Now you know what to eat, but perhaps you're perplexed about how it all fits together. These sample meal plans, which use recommendations from MyPyramid, give you an idea of how the process works.

1,600 Calories

Breakfast

1 cup whole-grain cereal
1 cup 1% low-fat milk
Half of a medium banana

Snack

Half of a medium banana
1 teaspoon peanut or almond butter

Lunch

2 ounces boneless, skinless chicken
1 teaspoon reduced-calorie mayonnaise

2 slices whole-grain bread
12 baby carrots
8 ounces fat-free or 1% low-fat milk

Snack

1½ ounces hard cheese, such as cheddar
1 mini (1 ounce) whole-grain bagel

Dinner

3 ounces cooked salmon, pork tenderloin, or lean beef
½ cup cooked rice with 1 teaspoon trans fat–free tub margarine
1 cup cooked broccoli with 1 teaspoon trans fat–free tub margarine
   or olive oil

Snack

8 ounces fruit-flavored, fat-free yogurt
1 medium apple
Discretionary calories: 132

2,400 Calories

Breakfast

1 cup whole-grain cereal
1 cup fat-free or 1% low-fat milk
1 slice whole-grain toast with 2 teaspoons trans fat–free tub margarine
Half of a medium banana

Snack

Half of a medium banana
1 teaspoon peanut or almond butter

Lunch

Salad: 2 ounces cooked boneless, skinless chicken or turkey; 2 cups
   dark leafy green vegetables; ½ cup canned, drained beans, such as
   black beans; ½ cup chopped tomato. Top with 2 teaspoons olive oil
   and balsamic vinegar.

1 2-ounce whole-grain roll
8 ounces fruit-flavored, fat-free yogurt
1 medium pear, apple, or orange

Snack

1½ ounces hard cheese, such as cheddar
7 soda crackers
12 baby carrots

Dinner

4 ounces cooked salmon, pork tenderloin, or lean beef
½ cup cooked rice with 1 teaspoon trans fat–free tub margarine
1 cup cooked broccoli with 1 teaspoon trans fat–free tub margarine
    or olive oil
1 cup cooked carrots

Snack

3 cups low-fat popcorn, popped
Discretionary calories: 362

Timing Is Everything

Is it better to eat six times a day or three? Will you gain weight if you consume most of your calories in the evening? What's the best way to eat to maximize energy? These are common questions and valid concerns, especially when you're pregnant or contemplating pregnancy, breast-feeding, or trying to shed pounds.

It's best to spread out meals and snacks during the day to provide your body with the energy it needs; eating three to six meals is fine, as long as you adhere to your calorie allowance. Pregnant and nursing women will need to eat often, given the energy demands made on their bodies.

You won't automatically gain weight by leaving the bulk of your calories until evening, but you might overeat. When you're too tired to police yourself, it's easier to lose control of the calories you're consuming.

Superfoods for Expectant Mothers

All foods are good, but some foods are better than others. MyPyramid encourages nutrient-dense foods because they provide more nutrients for the calories than other, similar foods. The following foods are among the most nutrient-dense superfoods for moms and expectant mothers. You'll find recipes for these and other fantastic foods in chapter 8.

Beef: Beef is rich in protein; the B vitamins niacin (vitamin B_3), B_6, and B_{12}; and zinc and iron in highly absorbable forms. Beef is also an excellent source of choline, which is required for proper brain development and for preventing neural tube defects. Add lean ground beef to pasta sauces; use it in tacos, for burgers, in stir-fry dishes, and in chili. Use lean cuts of beef for soups and stews.

Berries: The small size of berries belies their nutritional prowess. Berries are rich in potassium, folate, fiber, fluid, carbohydrates, and vitamin C. The phytonutrients in berries protect cells from damage. Top a whole-grain cereal with berries; use berries in smoothies made with yogurt or milk, in pancakes and other quick breads, and in salads; and eat plain as a snack.

Broccoli: Broccoli provides folate, fiber, and calcium; lutein, zeaxanthin, and carotenoids (which bolster vision); and potassium (for fluid balance and normal blood pressure). Broccoli also contains the raw materials for vitamin A production in your body and your baby's body. Add broccoli to pasta and stir-fry dishes; enjoy it steamed and topped with a smattering of olive oil; puree cooked broccoli and add to soups. Lightly coat bite-size pieces with olive oil and roast for about fifteen minutes on a baking sheet at 400°F until tender.

Cheese: Cheese supplies concentrated amounts of calcium and magnesium (for your bones and your baby's bones) as well as vitamin B_{12} and protein. Reduced-fat varieties, such as cheddar and part-skim mozzarella, save on calories, fat, and cholesterol. Eat cheese as a snack with whole-grain crackers or fruit; sprinkle grated cheese on top of soups; and add cheese to salads, sandwiches, and omelets.

Eggs: Eggs are the gold standard of protein because they provide all of the amino acids that you and your baby need to thrive.

They include more than a dozen vitamins and minerals as well as other nutrients, including choline (for brain development and preventing birth defects) and lutein and zeaxanthin (for healthy eyesight). Certain brands of eggs supply more of the omega-3 fats that your baby needs for proper brain development and peak vision; check the label to be sure you're getting docosahexaenoic acid (DHA) for the most benefit. Enjoy eggs in omelets and frittatas; hard-cooked in salads and sandwiches or as a snack; and as part of homemade waffles, crepes, and whole-grain French toast.

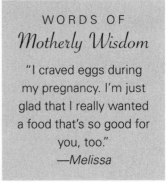

WORDS OF
Motherly Wisdom

"I craved eggs during my pregnancy. I'm just glad that I really wanted a food that's so good for you, too."
—*Melissa*

Legumes: Chickpeas, lentils, black beans, soybeans, and other beans supply fiber, protein, iron, folate, calcium, and zinc. Use them in chili, soups, salads, and pasta dishes; as hummus with whole-grain crackers; and as a filling in roll-up sandwiches.

Milk: Milk is an excellent source of calcium, phosphorus, and vitamin D—bone-building nutrients that a mother and her child require every day. Milk is also rich in protein, vitamin A, and several B vitamins. Drink plain or flavored milk; use it to make hot chocolate; include it in smoothies made with fruit; top whole-grain cereal and fruit with it; and use it in pudding. Prepare oatmeal in the microwave with milk instead of water to work in a serving of dairy.

Orange juice: 100% orange juice is an excellent choice of fruit juice because it supplies hefty doses of vitamin C, potassium, and folate, which is necessary for preventing certain birth defects. Orange juice with added calcium and vitamin D contains the same levels of these nutrients as milk does. Have a glass of it at breakfast or at any time of day; freeze OJ as pops or ice cubes; and use it in smoothies.

Pork tenderloin: Are you tired of chicken? Pork tenderloin is leaner than skinless chicken breast. Pork supplies several B vitamins as well as protein, iron, zinc, and choline. Grill, broil, or bake pork tenderloin.

Salmon: Salmon supplies high-quality protein to you and your baby. It's also an excellent source of omega-3 fats, which are necessary for peak brain development and vision in developing babies and in newborns. Grill or broil salmon, and use canned salmon in salads, sandwiches, burgers, and pasta dishes. Eat no more than twelve ounces of salmon (or other seafood considered safe during the childbearing years) each week. See chapter 6 for more on seafood safety.

Sweet potato: Sweet potatoes provide vitamin C, folate, fiber, and carotenoids (compounds that your body converts to vitamin A). Sweet potatoes also supply potassium in large amounts. They are delicious baked and cold as snacks and as side dishes. Mash cooked, peeled sweet potatoeswith orange juice, or roast them as follows: slice washed sweet potatoes into wedges, coat lightly with canola oil, and roast on a baking sheet at 400°F until tender, fifteen to twenty minutes.

Whole grains: Whole grains contain more fiber and trace nutrients than do processed grains like white rice and white flour. Enriched whole grains are fortified with folic acid and other B vitamins, iron, and zinc. Have some oatmeal for breakfast; use whole-grain breads for sandwiches; make brown rice, wild rice, whole-wheat pasta (including whole-wheat couscous), or quinoa for dinner; and snack on popcorn or whole-grain crackers.

Yogurt (plain, low-fat or fat-free): Yogurt supplies protein, calcium, B vitamins, and zinc; some brands also supply vitamin D, so check the label. Plain yogurt contains more calcium than milk does. Combine plain yogurt with fruit preserves or honey, fresh or dried fruit, or crunchy whole-grain cereal. Use plain or vanilla yogurt to top cooked sweet potatoes or for smoothies.

Moving On

You should now have an idea of an eating plan that suits you, whether you are waiting for pregnancy, are expecting, or are nursing. You can see from MyPyramid's organization that each food group supplies important nutrients and that all of the food groups work together to provide balance.

Don't expect perfection when you use MyPyramid or any other plan for a healthy diet. The idea is to come as close as possible to MyPyramid's suggested servings while incorporating a variety of foods in your eating plan. It may take some practice, so have fun working with it.

The next chapter delves into pregnancy and all its stages. You'll learn about what your body is going through or will go through, how your baby develops, and what to expect on the nine-month journey to delivery.

4

Pregnancy: Expect the Best

Hooray! You're pregnant. Maybe you've waited for this baby for a long time—or perhaps you weren't anticipating pregnancy so soon. Whatever the case, healthy living and regular visits to a licensed health-care professional (such as a doctor or a certified nurse-midwife) are now the ticket for having the healthiest child possible.

The First Trimester (Weeks 1 to 13)

What's Going On in There?

Your pregnancy may not yet be obvious to others, but you're certainly feeling the effects. An abundance of pregnancy hormones that support implantation, the growth of the uterus and the placenta, and the expansion of your circulatory system during early pregnancy leave you with constant reminders that you're expecting.

During early pregnancy, common experiences include tender breasts, frequent urination, rapid changes in blood pressure, extreme emotions, bouts of unexpected fatigue, intense hunger, a heightened sensitivity to smells, and so-called morning sickness that can last all day. Of course, you won't experience all of these, and even when you do experience pregnancy side effects, they can be mild. However you feel, what's happening in the womb at this point sets the stage for your child's well-being for life.

After the sperm meets up with the egg, about six days pass before the embryo implants itself in the uterine lining. Once an embryo has secured itself in the womb, it starts receiving blood and nutrition from the mother. The cells of the embryo, which are multiplying at breakneck speed, begin to differentiate (that is, develop specific functions) soon after implantation. The process of differentiation produces specialized cells that organize themselves into tissues and organs, such as the brain, the heart, the liver, and the circulatory system.

Tissues and organs develop on a tight timetable, but they don't all take shape at the same rate during these thirteen weeks. However, by the time the second trimester starts, all cell differentiation is complete. That's why it's so important for you to avoid nutritional deficiencies, particularly of folic acid, and substances that are harmful to organ development during this time (and throughout pregnancy), including alcohol, certain medications, and all recreational (illicit) drugs, such as marijuana and cocaine. It's also critical to avoid serious infections, such as rubella (German measles), radiation from X-rays or radiation therapy, and toxic contaminants, including mercury and lead.

How Much to Eat Now

You're eating for two, but that doesn't mean you should double the calories. In fact, you don't need any extra calories yet. There's no need to eat more, because the baby is so small—weighing only about an ounce by the end of the first trimester—and fetal growth, though rapid, does not yet require any additional energy. However, the daily quotas for several important nutrients, including folic acid, increase dramatically. That's why it's so important to make wise food choices during this time.

Stick with your personalized MyPyramid Prepregnancy Plan until the second trimester, using it as a guide for making healthy food choices. (If you've just received the good news that you're expecting, see chapter 3 for how to proceed with a healthy eating plan.)

Although you don't actually need to eat more, if you feel hungrier than usual during the first trimester, there's no reason to deprive yourself of food, as long as you're making healthy choices most of the time. Avoid using your pregnancy as a reason to overeat or to choose low-nutrient, high-fat foods over more nutritious fare, however. If you were trying to drop some pounds before pregnancy, put off that goal until after delivery. Pregnancy is no time to try to lose weight.

Some women who have dealt with an eating disorder in the past, or who are struggling with one when they conceive, may be fearful of gaining weight during pregnancy. It's important to discuss your feelings about food with qualified health-care professionals. It might be worthwhile to speak with a mental health professional and a registered dietitian (RD) who specializes in eating disorders.

If you're pregnant with twins, triplets, or more, don't wait until the second trimester to boost your calorie intake; you need to increase your calorie consumption right away. Aim to add 500 calories a day to your MyPyramid Prepregnancy Plan as soon as you find out you're having more than one baby. Your pregnancy probably won't be full-term—twins are typically born at about the thirty-fifth week and triplets often even earlier—and the goal is to maximize weight gain early in the pregnancy. Research suggests that the amount of weight you put on prior to the twentieth week of pregnancy influences your babies' growth before and after that time, and a greater weight can help to lengthen your pregnancy, bringing it closer to forty weeks.

Expect to gain two to five pounds during the first trimester, and possibly more with twins. You might not gain anything if you've been queasy for weeks on end, however. Your health-care provider will weigh you at your first prenatal visit and at every visit until delivery. By recording your weight on a regular basis, your health-care provider gauges whether you're putting on the right number of pounds to promote a healthy birth weight. Recording your weight is also useful for monitoring large decreases or increases in weight that could signal a problem.

There's probably no need to weigh yourself often at home, because a pregnant woman's weight can fluctuate due to fluid gains and losses, and these changes have little to do with overall weight gain.

WORDS OF
Motherly Wisdom

"I was worried about getting headaches from giving up caffeine, but I found that the slightest scent of coffee was enough to make me nauseous when I was pregnant. I didn't even want coffee, and I didn't get any headaches, either."
—*Robin*

Taking Care of Yourself

If you haven't already done so, stop smoking cigarettes and quit alcohol and recreational drugs. Substance abuse during pregnancy increases the risk of low-birth-weight and preterm infants, as well as other problems.

Steer clear of all topical and oral acne treatments that contain vitamin A or its derivatives, including Accutane, Retin-A, and Renova. However, do not automatically stop taking medications that treat chronic conditions, including depression, asthma, diabetes, and thyroid disease. Tell the physicians who help you to manage these conditions about your pregnancy, so you can proceed in the safest manner. In fact, check every medication you take with your doctor or pharmacist for its safety during pregnancy, including over-the-counter painkillers and anti-inflammatory drugs such as ibuprofen.

> WORDS OF
> *Motherly Wisdom*
>
> "When I was at work, I would close the door to my office and nap. It worked like a charm to boost my energy during all three of my pregnancies."
> —*Sarah*

Try as much as you can to pamper yourself and avoid unnecessary stress like additional responsibilities at work or huge home renovation projects. Ask for help, and allow your spouse or partner and others to shoulder some of the responsibility of cooking and cleaning. Get plenty of sleep and rest when you can, even if it means putting your head down on your desk at work to take a catnap during your lunch hour.

Eating Less but Still Gaining Weight

You're nauseated nearly all day long. You can't stand the sight or smell of most of your favorite foods. It's tough to even remember when you last ate a decent meal. Nevertheless, you're gaining weight. What gives?

It's possible to put on pounds during the first trimester even when your appetite has seemingly disappeared. Pregnancy hormones promote fluid retention, which can be responsible for some weight gain. You might also be less active than normal, which could be responsible for the rest of the weight gain.

Do You Need a Prenatal Supplement?

Most women receive a prescription for prenatal vitamin and mineral supplements immediately after a positive pregnancy test. Because prescribing prenatal vitamin pills is the common practice, you might be surprised to learn that that it could be unnecessary. There is no official expert opinion that all women need the nutrients in prescription prenatal pills in the doses they provide. (Iron is the possible exception.)

Vitamin and mineral pills (multis) are not substitutes for a healthy diet at any time of life. However, they are capable of filling gaps for important nutrients, such as folic acid, that promote good health for you and your growing child. It's a good idea to take at least a daily multi with close to 100 percent of the Daily Value (DV) for iron and folic acid prior to and during pregnancy, throughout breast-feeding, and afterward.

Choose a multi with mostly beta-carotene as the source of vitamin A, and do not exceed 3,000 micrograms (mcg) or 10,000 International Units (IU) a day in supplemental vitamin A. If your multi supplies less than 600 mcg of folic acid, which is the recommended amount for pregnancy, be sure to include one or more servings a day of foods that are fortified with folic acid, such as breakfast cereal, pasta, and rice. Your daily multi should provide 100 percent of the DV for iron and at least 200 mg DHA.

If your diet was poor at the outset of your pregnancy or at any time during it, or if your diet had been inadequate for months prior to conception, you're probably a good candidate for a daily prescription prenatal pill, which supplies nutrients in much higher amounts than over-the-counter multis. Women who are carrying more than one baby will benefit from a prescription prenatal supplement with DHA, and so will those with certain chronic conditions such as diabetes. Women who have had a pregnancy affected by a neural tube defect such as spina bifida should speak with their doctor before conception for prescription-level doses of folic acid. When you begin the supplements your doctor has prescribed, cease taking your daily multivitamin.

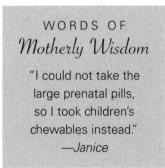

WORDS OF
Motherly Wisdom

"I could not take the large prenatal pills, so I took children's chewables instead."
—Janice

All about Iron

Iron needs increase significantly during pregnancy as your body produces more red blood cells to support your growing baby, depleting the supply of stored iron in your body. Even with a healthy diet, it's nearly impossible for most women to reach their daily iron quota of 27 mg during pregnancy. The Centers for Disease Control and Prevention recommends that all pregnant women start taking a low-dose iron supplement of 30 mg at the first prenatal visit, either as an individual supplement or in a prenatal vitamin. Most prenatal vitamins contain 27 to 60 mg of iron. After testing your blood, your doctor may recommend even more iron, often 60 to 120 mg a day, in addition to a prenatal vitamin.

Although some experts contend that it's not necessary to take large doses of iron if you are not iron-deficient, many women are low in iron well before conception, so extra iron during pregnancy typically makes sense. There is rarely a need to take prescription-strength prenatal pills before conceiving or after delivery, however.

Problems with Prenatal Pills

It's possible that you won't be able to tolerate the pills your doctor has prescribed, because of either the large size or the high levels of iron, which can cause an upset stomach, diarrhea, or constipation. Tell your health-care provider if you are not taking the pills he or she has prescribed. You might be able to switch to a smaller prenatal pill with less iron, pills with a slicker coating to make them go down more easily, a regular multi, or a chewable vitamin with iron. If constipation is troubling you, follow a high-fiber diet with plenty of fluids. Take your pill at night or after meals to avoid queasiness, or cut it in half to split up the dosage during the day.

Do-It-Yourself Supplements

Many women choose to forgo prescription prenatal supplements for the over-the-counter variety. There is no set formula for what should be in prenatal supplements, so you'll have to figure out on your own what to take and what to avoid. The following table, from the Institute of Medicine, is meant to guide your choice of a supplement for pregnancy and nursing. (Teens may need more of some of the nutrients listed here. See chapter 3 for specific needs.)

DAILY VITAMIN AND MINERAL NEEDS

Nutrient	Pregnancy (19–50 years old)	Lactation (19–50 years old)
Vitamin A*, mcg	770 (2,541IU)	1,300 (4,290 IU)
Vitamin C, mg	85	120
Vitamin D, IU	200 (5mcg)	200 (5mcg)
Vitamin E, IU	22 (15mg)	28 (19mg)
Vitamin K, mcg	90	90
Vitamin B_1 (thiamin), mg	1.4	1.4
Vitamin B_2 (riboflavin), mg	1.4	1.6
Vitamin B_3 (niacin), mg	18	17
Vitamin B_5 (pantothenic acid), mg	6	7
Vitamin B_6, mg	1.9	2
Folate, mcg	600	500
Choline, mcg	450	550
Vitamin B_{12}, mcg	2.6	2.8
Calcium**, mg	1,000	1,000
Iodine, mcg	220	290
Iron, mg	27	9
Magnesium, mg	350	310
Zinc, mg	11	12

Mcg = micrograms, mg = milligrams, and IU = International Units.

*Choose a supplement with most of the vitamin A as beta-carotene. Do not exceed 3,000 IU of vitamin A on a daily basis during pregnancy.

**Multis are generally low in calcium, so you may need a separate calcium supplement if you don't get enough calcium from foods.

Food and Daily Values

Many foods are fortified with the nutrients you need when you are expecting a child and when you are breast-feeding. In fact, the food supply is so heavily fortified that you could consume excessive amounts of certain nutrients, especially if you are also taking a multivitamin or a prescription prenatal vitamin pill, which supplies at least 100 percent, and often far more, of your daily needs.

To know what you're getting from foods and dietary supplements, use the information about nutrients that is expressed in the percentage of DV on food and supplement labels. DVs provide a basis for determining how one serving of that food or supplement fits into your daily requirements. There is one tiny glitch, however: the DV percentage is based on a 2,000-calorie diet for adults older than eighteen and is not meant for pregnant and nursing women. It doesn't matter; DVs are still the best guideline there is for making choices about foods and supplements.

Here is a list of the DVs used on food labels.

Nutrient	Daily Value (DV)
Vitamin A	5,000 IU
Vitamin C	60 mg
Vitamin B_1 (thiamin)	1.5 mg
Vitamin B_2 (riboflavin)	1.7 mg
Calcium	1,000 mg
Iron	18 mg
Vitamin D	400 IU
Vitamin E	30 IU
Vitamin B_6	2 mg
Folate or folic acid	400 mg
Vitamin B_{12}	6 mg
Iodine	150 mcg
Zinc	15 mg

Mcg = micrograms, mg = milligrams, and IU = International Units.

Simple math can help you to figure out nutrient content in a serving of food or a dietary supplement.

Example 1:

8 ounces of milk contains 30% DV for calcium
The DV for calcium is 1,000 mg
.30 × 1,000 mg = 300 mg
8 ounces of milk supplies 300 mg of calcium

Example 2:

1 cup of ready-to-eat cereal supplies 35% DV for iron
The DV for iron is 18 mg
.35 × 18 mg = 6.3 mg
1 cup of cereal provides 6.3 mg of iron

Nutritional Overkill

You can have too much of a good thing. For example, granola bars that are designed for pregnant and nursing women are often touted as providing all of the necessary supplemental nutrients for a normal pregnancy and for nursing, but they are actually more like a replacement for a daily multivitamin. A bar can contain at least 800 mcg of folic acid, which is 200 percent of the DV. Add this to the folic acid in your prescription prenatal pill (typically 1,000 mcg) and in the bowl of fortified cereal (400 mcg) you had for breakfast, and you'd be taking in at least 2,200 mcg of folic acid a day when you need only about one-fourth that amount.

DHA Supplements

Prenatal vitamins don't contain any fatty acids, including the beneficial omega-3 fats. DHA, an omega-3 fatty acid, is important for the development of your baby's brain, nerves, and eyes. The recommended intake of DHA during pregnancy and nursing is 200 to 300 mg a day—the amount you'd get if you ate five to ten ounces of cold-water fish, such as salmon or trout, every week—but few Americans get that much from their diet. It's very likely that you could benefit from a DHA supplement or DHA-fortified foods, such as those mentioned in chapter 2.

Outsmarting a Poor Appetite: Stealth Nutrition

Just a few weeks ago, in your prepregnancy life, you might have adored Chinese food, or perhaps you could not start your day without a cup of coffee. Now just the thought of these foods inspires a bout of nausea.

Food aversions—and their counterparts, food cravings (see the section on the second trimester in this chapter)—are most likely the result of pregnancy hormones. The hormonal surges that are brought on by pregnancy intensify your sense of smell, which heavily influences food preferences.

The only certainty about food aversions is their changeability. Food preferences tend to differ from pregnancy to pregnancy. That's why you might have loved sirloin

WORDS OF
Motherly Wisdom

"When I was having a hard time tolerating meat, I would whip up smoothies and add protein powder to them."
—*Meghan*

steak during your first pregnancy, but you can't bear the sight of it now. Even more puzzling is that food preferences can change on a daily basis. Pregnancy has even been known to alter a woman's preference for certain foods indefinitely.

Avoiding certain foods or entire food groups can become problematic, especially if you continue to shy away from them well into the second and third trimesters and you aren't making up for the nutrients (including calories, fat, and protein) that you're missing. The negative effects of food aversions on nutrient intake are intensified in the absence of a daily multiple vitamin and mineral dietary supplement.

Here are some tips for sneaking in the nutrition you may be missing:

- Stick with mild-tasting vegetables, such as mashed white or sweet potatoes, and green beans. Puree cooked legumes, such as canned garbanzo beans, and stronger-smelling vegetables, such as broccoli and cauliflower, and use as side dishes or sauces for meat. Warm foods are more aromatic, so work with cooked, cooled vegetables to keep nausea at bay.
- Whip up a fruit smoothie if you can't stand the thought of drinking milk or soy beverages, eating fruit; or both. Chapter 8 shows you how to prepare delicious, nutrient-packed drinks that are easy on the stomach.
- If meat is making you gag, turn to beans, soy, nuts, nut butters, and reduced-fat cheese for protein and other nutrients. For example, stir textured vegetable protein crumbles (made from soy) or low-sodium pureed cottage cheese into warm pasta sauce or add pureed, cooked canned and drained beans to soups and stews.
- Rely on eggs for protein, vitamins, and minerals. See chapter 8 for delicious and nutritious egg recipes.

Your Exercise Routine Now

There are so many good reasons to exercise; you can read all about them in chapter 1. When you're expecting, exercise has particular perks, including fewer aches and pains; less constipation, bloating, and swelling; improved energy level; stress reduction; and better sleep. Regular workouts during pregnancy can help you to cope better with labor and delivery, and they can also make it easier to get back in shape after your bundle of joy arrives.

Even better, according to the American College of Sports Medicine, exercise reduces the risk for preeclampsia, a condition of pregnancy that is marked by elevated blood pressure, protein in your urine, and dangerous swelling. Regular workouts help to prevent or manage gestational diabetes, the type of diabetes that first occurs during pregnancy; in some women, exercise can be enough to keep blood glucose levels under control.

Physical activity on a near-daily basis can also translate into a healthier birth weight. Researchers at Case Western Reserve University asked women who were eight weeks pregnant to either start exercising at a moderate pace three to five times a week or to do no exercise for the remainder of their pregnancies. The pregnant exercisers delivered infants who were significantly heavier and longer but still within a normal, healthy range for weight and length. The researchers concluded that regular exercise could be an easy way to boost a baby's growth during uncomplicated pregnancies, probably because physical activity encourages the flow of blood to the uterus.

As long as your health-care provider approves, you should exercise on a regular basis. Women with uncomplicated pregnancies need a minimum of thirty minutes of moderate activity on most days of the week. There's no need to overexert yourself to reap the rewards of working out, however. Exercising too vigorously can impede the flow of blood to your baby.

If you're just starting out, you might be more comfortable with programs that are specifically designed for pregnant women. You may already have a workout routine in place that you can continue, but you'll probably have to modify it at some point. You'll tire more easily now, so even the thirty-minute walk or the mile swim you've been doing all along could become challenging. No matter what activity you choose, always wear a bra that fits well and provides lots of support to help protect your breasts and make exercise comfortable. Invest in a new pair of comfortable sneakers and some loose-fitting workout gear, too.

Any Time Is a Good Time to Exercise

Even if you weren't working out before you conceived, you can start at any point in your pregnancy, as long your doctor says so. Now is not the time to take up a strenuous sport, however. In addition, there are some activities that you should put on hold until after delivery, even if you have been doing them for years (see "Do Not Try This at Home [or Anywhere Else!]" on page 107).

Walking is beneficial for most pregnant women, including beginners, because it's easy on the joints and the muscles. Swimming works several muscle groups at once and helps you to avoid injury; it also keeps you cool in hot weather. Cycling on a stationary bike avoids the risk of falling, which increases as pregnancy progresses. Strength training relieves tension and makes stronger muscles, which helps to prevent some of the aches and pains common in pregnancy. Aerobics is a good way to keep your heart and your lungs strong; as your pregnancy moves along, check out classes for pregnant women.

When exercise is part of your pregnancy routine, be sure to eat enough to satisfy your daily calorie quota. Even though calorie needs don't increase during the first trimester, you will need to recalculate your calorie requirements if you were sedentary before pregnancy and have begun working out on most days since conceiving.

Keep It Cool

A pregnant woman's body produces more heat because of a revved-up metabolism. In addition, working muscles generate heat that your body needs to release. The inability to get rid of heat can produce a dangerous spike in your core body temperature (normally 98.6°F) that could compromise your baby's brain development.

So-called overheating can be the result of exercising in a warm environment, such as a crowded aerobics room or gym, in hot and humid air, or in a combination of the two. Work out in cool, well-ventilated places and wear loose-fitting clothing. Avoid hot tubs, saunas, and whirlpools in order to keep heat to a minimum.

Inadequate fluid intake is another reason for overheating. Dehydration reduces blood volume and thus decreases the amount of oxygen-rich blood that flows to your baby. Pregnant women need thirteen cups of fluid daily; pregnant exercisers will need more. Drink plenty of fluid before, during, and after working out. When your urine is plentiful and very light in color, you have a normal fluid balance. If it's dark and scanty, you need more fluid.

> WORDS OF
> *Motherly Wisdom*
>
> "I swam when I was pregnant the second time around. I loved the feeling of weightlessness in the pool. I was in good shape going into delivery, and I bounced back faster than with my other pregnancies."
> —Meghan

When Exercise Is Off-Limits

It's hard to believe that exercise, with its myriad benefits, would ever be banned during pregnancy. There are some women who should not work out, however. According to the American College of Obstetricians and Gynecologists, women with the following conditions should avoid physical activity:

- Pregnancy-induced hypertension (high blood pressure).
- Preterm ruptured membranes (amniotic fluid leaks from the uterus); exercise can worsen this condition.
- Preterm labor in a previous or the current pregnancy (increases the chances of contractions).
- Insufficient cervical cerclage (the cervix dilates long before delivery); exercise can worsen this condition.
- Persistent second- or third-trimester bleeding; the placenta is attached abnormally to the uterus or is loose or separating.
- Intrauterine growth restriction (inability of the placenta to adequately nourish a growing baby); exercise can limit blood flow to the baby.

If you're dedicated to fitness, being told to discontinue your workouts can come as a blow. However, pregnancy is relatively short. You will soon be back to exercising after your bundle of joy arrives.

Do Not Try This at Home (or Anywhere Else!)

Working out is good for you, but certain activities are out of the question when you're expecting because of the potential risks to you and your child. Any activity involving pressure changes that could deprive a developing baby of oxygen and any sport with a high risk of falling or of abdominal trauma are inappropriate for pregnant women. Here's what *not* to do, even if you are a seasoned athlete or you've done these activities prior to pregnancy:

- Skydiving
- Surfing

> WORDS OF
> *Motherly Wisdom*
>
> "I'm a runner, and I thought I'd be able to continue during my third pregnancy, but I could only run until about the third month. I was just so tired that I chose sleep instead!"
> —Erin

- Kickboxing
- Scuba diving (snorkeling is okay)
- Downhill skiing or snowboarding (cross-country skiing is okay)
- Waterskiing
- Horseback riding
- Skateboarding
- Roller skating
- Ice skating
- Bike riding (stationary bikes are okay)
- Contact sports such as ice hockey, soccer, touch or tackle football, lacrosse, and basketball
- Gymnastics
- Hiking and mountain climbing
- Anything with jumping or jarring motions, such as high-impact aerobics classes

Know When to Say When

Stop exercising, and immediately call your doctor or other licensed health-care professional, if you experience any of the following:

- Chest pain
- Vaginal bleeding
- Fluid leaking from the vagina
- Dizziness or feelings of faintness
- Headache
- Decreased fetal movement (after the second trimester)
- Muscle weakness
- Calf pain or swelling
- Contractions
- Increased shortness of breath, difficulty breathing

WORDS OF
Motherly Wisdom

"I found out I was pregnant with my first child one week after completing my first marathon. Even though I was very fit, I was shocked by how quickly I got winded once I was pregnant. I cut back to walking, and I am so glad that I did. It worked out great for me."

—*Lisa*

Mitigating Miscarriage

Miscarriage, the spontaneous loss of a baby during the first half of pregnancy, typically takes place between the seventh and twelfth week. An estimated 10 to 15 percent of known pregnancies end in miscarriage. Since many miscarriages occur long before a woman realizes that she's expecting, the actual miscarriage rate could be much higher.

Women who have experienced three or more miscarriages run a greater risk of subsequent miscarriages, but don't let that alarm you. If you've had a miscarriage, it might be comforting for you to know that it's often a one-time event. Although a small percentage of women has had multiple miscarriages, more than 90 percent of pregnancies do not end that way. Finally, once the first trimester has passed, your chances for miscarrying plummet.

Nobody completely understands why miscarriages happen. However, experts say that most first-trimester pregnancies end on their own largely because of chromosomal abnormalities in the embryo or fetus. Too many or too few chromosomes can result in devastating developmental difficulties and death. Such miscarriages are not preventable. Second-trimester miscarriage (from thirteen to twenty weeks pregnant) is often caused by problems with the uterus or by a weakened cervix that dilates well before it should. As with first-trimester losses, chromosomal abnormalities are often culpable for these later miscarriages. Certain maternal immune-system problems (such as lupus) and other conditions, including infections and poorly controlled diabetes and thyroid disease, can also result in the second-trimester loss of a child.

The Effects of Time

Age influences miscarriage risk, in part because chromosomal abnormalities become more common with the passage of time. Miscarriage rates are higher in women thirty-five and older, but the father's age can matter, too. Miscarriage risk is highest when the mother is thirty-five or older and her partner is forty or older.

If you're in your mid-thirties and you're delaying pregnancy, you and your partner might want to get a move on it. If you are already pregnant, there's nothing you can do about your age, so there's no point in fretting about it. Instead, concentrate on how to bring your pregnancy to term. Start by seeking prenatal care as early in your pregnancy as possible and keeping regular appointments throughout your pregnancy.

Lifestyle

Mothers-to-be of any age can take heart in a study published in the *British Journal of Obstetrics and Gynaecology* that cited a number of lifestyle factors that lessen the likelihood of miscarriage. Among them are eating fruits and vegetables on a daily basis, taking vitamin supplements, experiencing nausea during pregnancy, and having previously delivered a child.

The researchers also found a link between the following factors and a higher risk of miscarriage: being underweight prior to conception, consuming alcohol regularly or in large amounts during pregnancy, having chronic stress, and the mother's having an older partner. Other research suggests that cigarette smoking and illicit (recreational) drugs are also associated with miscarriage. Caffeine can affect your chances, too, so to be on the safe side, curb your caffeine intake to 200 mg or less a day (see chapter 2).

The Second Trimester (Weeks 14 to 26)

What's Going On in There?

You'll probably feel your best during the second trimester; that's when a pregnant woman's energy typically returns. Many of the earlier effects of pregnancy subside during this trimester, including nausea, vomiting, and fatigue, but they do not all magically disappear once the fourteenth week begins.

As the second trimester of pregnancy proceeds, your baby measures about three inches, the size of your thumb. The face is well formed now, and the heart is beating with regularity. Your baby is capable of making a fist with fully formed fingers and can even engage in thumb sucking, if so inclined. Tooth buds that will eventually become primary teeth have appeared, and it's possible to tell on ultrasound whether you're having a boy or a girl.

The second trimester is when your child's growth begins in earnest. Bones, muscles, and organs become bigger and more developed. By the midpoint of your pregnancy—twenty weeks—your baby is about eight inches long. You might feel some turning, stretching, and kicking, starting around the sixteenth week. The heartbeat is stronger, so it's detectable with a stethoscope now. As the final trimester looms, an even more rapid development of the baby's brain and nervous system is on the horizon.

What to Eat Now

You need more food to fuel your baby's rapid growth. During the second trimester, that amounts to about 330 calories a day in women who started pregnancy at a healthy weight. Your basic eating plan won't change dramatically, however. Simply stick with your MyPyramid Prepregnancy Plan and add foods from the five food groups.

If you have not done so, see chapter 3 to determine the appropriate MyPyramid Prepregnancy Plan for yourself and make the wisest food choices for you and your child.

Weight Gain

Even with the guidelines, it's difficult to determine the exact number of calories a pregnant woman needs to gain the right amount of weight. That's because calorie needs are personal. As long as you're gaining adequate weight on a steady basis on a healthy diet, you're probably eating enough.

Eating extra calories means that you'll be piling on the pounds during the next nine months. If you have spent years trying to stave off extra body fat, gaining weight probably does not sit well with you, in spite of the excitement you feel about your impending arrival. However, gaining weight during pregnancy is for a very good cause—the health of your baby.

How Much Weight Should You Gain?

The number of pounds you should put on when you're expecting depends on your prepregnancy body mass index (BMI) and on how many babies you're carrying. If you haven't already done so, see chapter 1 to learn how to calculate your body mass using your body weight prior to conception.

Gaining extra weight won't necessarily mean you'll have a bigger baby, but it could mean more body fat for you that is difficult to drop after delivery. Gaining too few pounds, however, is risky to the development of your child's full physical and mental potential. The proper amount of weight gain continues to be important after the second trimester, too; low weight gain during the third trimester is linked to a greater risk of preterm delivery. The following list tells you how much weight you should gain based on your preconception BMI.

If your BMI was . . .	Gain this much weight . . .
Less than 19.8	28 to 40 pounds
19.8 to 26.0	25 to 35 pounds
26.1 to 29.0	15 to 25 pounds
Greater than 29.0	At least 15 pounds
Twin pregnancy, any BMI	35 to 45 pounds

Does Birth Weight Determine Destiny?

Birth weight is a good indicator of a baby's overall health at birth and beyond. The size of your baby on delivery day is largely up to you, because your pregnancy weight gain will strongly influence the delivery weight. Gaining the recommended number of pounds for your prepregnancy body mass does not always translate into a perfectly healthy child, but it's a huge step in the right direction.

Infants born to women who gain weight within the suggested range typically require fewer medical interventions after delivery, whereas children born to women who gain too little weight tend to be undersized and more likely to arrive before thirty-seven weeks. In addition to needing specialized medical care early in life, underweight babies (those weighing five and a half pounds or less) also run a greater risk of developing certain chronic conditions as young children and adults, including obesity, diabetes, high blood pressure, and heart disease.

Adequate weight gain also influences the mother's health during pregnancy. If you put on more than thirty-five pounds, there's a greater risk for developing preeclampsia than if weight gain is less than thirty-five pounds. Being overweight at conception and gaining more than the recommended number of pounds during pregnancy increases the likelihood of impaired glucose tolerance (higher than normal blood glucose levels). It also increases your chances of a cesarean delivery and makes it harder to return to a healthy weight after the baby is born.

Starting Pregnancy with Extra Pounds

Beginning a pregnancy when you're overweight increases the chances of complications for both mother and child. The more overweight you are, the harder the pregnancy will be on you and your baby. If you're already pregnant, there's not much you can do now—or is there?

When researchers from the St. Louis University School of Medicine surveyed the results of the pregnancies of 120,000 obese women (defined as having a BMI of at least 30) who gained no more than fifteen pounds during pregnancy, they found that the risk of preeclampsia, cesarean delivery, and delivering larger children decreased. Some women delivered underweight babies, however.

In a study of ninety-six obese women with gestational diabetes, researchers from the same medical school found that calorie restriction and exercise during pregnancy resulted in more babies of normal birth weight without any negative effects. Babies born to women who lost weight or maintained their weight while pregnant were more likely to be of normal size.

If you're overweight and pregnant, do not put yourself on a diet. Ask your health-care provider how much weight you should gain, then stick with that recommendation.

Timing Matters

When you gain weight during pregnancy is just as important as *how much* you gain. Perhaps you added just a few pounds to your frame during the first trimester. For the rest of the pregnancy, gaining weight on a steady basis is a must.

Once the first trimester has passed, plan to add a pound or so each week, or about four pounds per month. Overweight women (those starting pregnancy at a BMI of above 26) should put on about two-thirds of a pound weekly, or nearly three pounds per month. Underweight women, those with a BMI at or below 19.8 at conception, need to gain slightly more than a pound each week, or about four to five pounds monthly. Women pregnant with more than one fetus should gain about one and a half pounds each week, for a total of six pounds each month.

You might not gain exactly according to the weekly guidelines, however. For example, women with a multiple pregnancy may experience more nausea and vomiting than other pregnant women, so weight gain could be more difficult; also, a multiple pregnancy is usually shorter—about thirty-five weeks rather than forty. That's not necessarily a problem, as long as you gain the suggested amount for the month. However, if you consistently gain too little or too much weight from one doctor's visit to the next, it can be a sign that your diet should be adjusted or that you have another problem.

If you're gaining weight too fast, review the suggested eating pattern in your MyPyramid Pregnancy Plan and see how closely you're adhering to it. You may need to adjust portion sizes; choose foods with less fat, like grilled chicken instead of fried or 1% low-fat milk instead of whole; or both. Check your diet for excessively salty foods, such as canned soups and other processed and fast foods, including pizza, to see whether sodium-packed foods are to blame. Women who have excessive weight gain during pregnancy shouldn't attempt to lose what they have put on, but they should try to bring their rate of gain within a healthy range.

Inadequate weight gain during pregnancy is most likely due to not eating enough. You may need to recalculate your calorie needs according to MyPyramid, then be sure to include all of the recommended servings every day. Persistent nausea and vomiting, which can last for an entire pregnancy, may be another reason for lower-than-desired calorie intake. Intentionally restricting calories to keep weight gain low can harm your baby's growth and development.

Women who gain too much weight or not enough weight for any reason during their pregnancies would benefit from the advice of an RD, who can tailor an eating plan that's right for them.

Where the Pounds Go

Your girth is expanding, and you'd like to know where all that extra weight is going. Only about one-third of the weight you gain is actually the baby. Here's a list that tells exactly where your pregnancy pounds go:

Baby: 7 to 8 pounds
Placenta: 1 to 2 pounds
Amniotic fluid: 2 pounds
Breasts: 1 pound
Uterus: 2 pounds
Increased blood volume: 3 pounds
Body fat: 5 or more pounds
Increased muscle tissue and fluid: 4 to 7 pounds
Total: At least 25 pounds

Managing Pregnancy Cravings

Once the first trimester is over, your appetite may return with a vengeance! You've probably heard tales of loved ones being dispatched at all hours to search for a certain brand of bacon double cheeseburger or Rocky Road ice cream to quell an expectant mother's desire. Now you're the one who's feeling an overwhelming urge to splurge.

Intense longings for salt-laden chips, stuffed-crust pizza, and double chocolate chip cookies are most likely being driven by pregnancy hormones. Craving certain foods and eating them can also be how you comfort yourself when you're tired or crabby.

Food cravings get a bad rap, sometimes with good reason. A 2007 *British Journal of Nutrition* study found that pregnant women who feast on so-called junk food may have children with a propensity for becoming overweight later in life, which supports the notion that it's possible to program a child's preferences for high-fat fare while the child is still in the womb.

In the study, pregnant and nursing laboratory rats consumed regular lab chow or a steady diet of biscuits, marshmallows, jam, doughnuts, potato chips, and candy bars. The rats whose mothers ate the junk-food diet while they were pregnant and nursing put on more weight after birth than the rats born to mothers who consumed rat chow. It seems that the baby rats were less able to switch off their appetites and stop eating even when they had consumed enough calories, making them prone to putting on excess weight. Nobody is sure why this happened, but high levels of sugar or fat in the blood before birth can alter the development

WORDS OF
Motherly Wisdom

"After having avoided meat for nearly seven years, I had unbelievable and undeniable cravings for red meat during my first pregnancy. I could not get enough! But my other two pregnancies didn't have the same effect. In fact, with my third, I had very little appetite—at least at first."
—*Lisa*

Keep Cravings Safe

No matter how strong the craving is, don't give in to eating raw or undercooked seafood (including sushi and sashimi), meat, and eggs; unpasteurized juice and unpasteurized milk and foods made from the latter, including Brie, feta, Camembert, Roquefort, and Mexican-style cheeses; raw vegetable sprouts, including alfalfa, clover, and radish; certain herbal teas not sold in the supermarket; and alcohol. These and other foods are more likely to make you sick during pregnancy or endanger the growth and development of your baby. See chapter 6 for more on food safety.

of the fat cells as well as the pathways in the brain that regulate hunger and feelings of fullness.

Eating too much of any food, healthy or otherwise, during pregnancy may lead to excessive weight gain that boosts the risk for complications, including gestational diabetes and high blood pressure. Don't forget to figure in the calories from between-meal indulgences.

A steady diet of high-fat, low-nutrient snacks adds insult to injury. Snack chips, french fries, and soft drinks often replace foods that offer more nutrition for you and your baby. You do not have to give up snacking or eating the foods you crave, but controlling pregnancy cravings will be easier with the following strategies:

- Eat on a regular basis to prevent intense hunger that can trigger cravings.
- Make sure that your meals include protein, carbohydrates, and some fat.
- Consider your hunger level. Maybe you just need a short break to relieve stress.
- Go ahead and indulge—in small amounts. Try eating less than you normally would. For example, when you can't resist chips, choose a one-ounce bag of the baked variety instead of a large bag of the fried ones.

When cravings strike before, during, or after pregnancy, reach for the following healthier options:

Crunchy. Instead of chips or some other equally fattening food, try one of these options: flavored rice cakes; chips made from toasted whole-wheat pita bread and sprinkled with grated Parmesan cheese; an ounce of nuts or sunflower seeds; low-fat popcorn; an ounce of reduced-fat cheese, such as cheddar, and six whole-grain crackers; ten small whole-grain pretzels topped with a tablespoon of almond or peanut butter; a quarter cup of trail mix (equal parts whole-grain cereal, chopped nuts, dried fruit, sunflower seeds, and miniature chocolate chips); or raw carrots or celery.

Creamy. Instead of a big bowl of ice cream, reach for one of the following: a 100-calorie cup of low-fat ice cream; eight ounces of low-fat vanilla, coffee, or fruit-flavored yogurt; or a smoothie made with fruit and yogurt.

Chocolate. Put down the king-size chocolate bar and choose one of these instead: chocolate pudding prepared with low-fat milk; a 100-calorie frozen fudge bar; hot chocolate or chocolate milk made with low-fat milk; chocolate-dipped strawberries or dried fruit; or a choco-banana frappe made with one cup of 1% low-fat chocolate milk, one medium banana, and two ice cubes.

Sweet. Skip the pastry and have one of these healthier options: two graham crackers spread with low-fat cream cheese and strawberry jam; half a whole-wheat bagel spread with peanut butter and drizzled with honey; six small or two large rice cakes spread with one-half cup of part-skim ricotta cheese and sprinkled with a quarter teaspoon of sugar and a pinch of ground cinnamon; angel food cake drizzled with fat-free chocolate sauce; frozen pops made with 100% orange juice; sorbet; sherbet; frozen fruit; or dried fruit.

Pica: Cravings Gone Wrong

Pica is the name for the cravings that some pregnant women have for nonfood items, including dirt, clay, paper, and even paint chips. No one knows exactly why pica happens, but it can signal an iron deficiency. Expectant mothers may also get the urge to eat raw flour or cornstarch, which, despite being food items, are a problem in large amounts; too much can lead to blocked bowels and can replace essential nutrients in your diet by causing feelings of fullness. If you have the urge to eat nonfood items, report them to your doctor immediately.

Coping with Stress

Stress is part of our daily lives. Some stress is considered beneficial because it motivates us to get things done. Persistent, severe stress is not good, however, especially when you're pregnant. Divorce, the death of a loved one, a job loss, worry about your relationship with your baby's father, or financial woes are all sources of stress that can be detrimental to you and your child.

High levels of ongoing stress can result in fatigue, sleeplessness, poor appetite, and headaches, among other side effects. In some cases, severe stress boosts the risk of preterm birth.

Poor nutrition makes it more difficult to deal with stress, whether you're pregnant or not. Eating a healthy diet and taking a multivitamin every day can provide some of the stamina you need to deal with constant stress. Regular physical activity, as long as it has been approved by your doctor, relieves stress, too.

Preeclampsia

Preeclampsia is a potentially dangerous condition that can develop quickly in the second trimester or later in pregnancy. Preeclampsia is marked by elevated blood pressure, swelling due to fluid retention, and abnormal kidney function that results in protein spilling into the urine. See chapter 7 for the details of preeclampsia and how to prevent it with diet and a healthy lifestyle.

Food Allergies

Food allergies are frightening and potentially deadly, so you will want to do everything possible to prevent your child from becoming intolerant to milk, eggs, peanuts, tree nuts (such as walnuts and almonds), seafood, soy, or wheat, the foods that account for 90 percent of all food-allergic reactions. What you eat during pregnancy (and nursing) could affect the incidence of food allergies in your child.

Food allergies are a hyperreaction to the proteins in foods called *allergens*. When you have a food allergy, the body's immune system interprets food allergens as threats and sets in motion a cascade of events to get rid of the so-called invaders. Food allergens cannot be disarmed with cooking or through digestion.

If you, your partner, or one of your children has a food allergy, your future children are more prone to have one, too. You may have heard that it's possible to reduce the risk of a food allergy in your child by avoiding highly allergenic foods, such as peanuts, during pregnancy or breast-feeding. A 2008 report from the American Academy of Pediatrics, which once endorsed the avoidance of allergens during pregnancy and nursing, now says that this practice is probably unnecessary. The study does point out some evidence that avoiding certain foods when you're breast-feeding can reduce the risk of your child developing eczema, but the likelihood of that happening depends on your family history. The report also points out the following:

- Soy-based infant formulas do not seem to help prevent allergies.
- There's no reason to wait, with the idea of preventing allergies, beyond four to six months to start babies on solid food.
- Although breast-feeding is an excellent way to help build your child's immune system, exclusive breast-feeding does not appear to protect babies from allergic asthma that starts after the age of six or so.
- Speak with your doctor about your family's history of allergies and asthma to determine how to proceed with your diet when you're expecting or nursing. If you eliminate an entire food group, speak with an RD to make sure that you're getting the nutrients you need for yourself and your child.

Allergy or Intolerance?

An intolerance to a certain food is sometimes misinterpreted as a food allergy. For example, lactose intolerance, the inability of the body to break down lactose, the natural carbohydrate in milk, is not a milk allergy because it does not involve the immune system. The symptoms of lactose intolerance, including gas, bloating, and diarrhea, are uncomfortable, but they are fleeting and don't cause lasting harm. Ask your doctor or an allergist about any adverse reactions you have to a food in order to be sure of the difference between a food allergy and a food intolerance.

Exercise During the Second Trimester: Keep Moving

By the second trimester, you might finally be feeling energetic again. Take advantage of this newfound get-up-and-go and start working out, if you haven't been doing so already. As always, ask your doctor what type of physical activity is best for you, even if you have been exercising since the beginning of your pregnancy. Exercise can be dangerous for women with pregnancy-induced high blood pressure or other conditions covered earlier in this chapter. Make sure you're eating the right amount of food to keep your weight gain on track.

For the previous thirteen weeks, your blood levels of pregnancy hormones, particularly progesterone, have been on the rise. That's beneficial, because progesterone preps your body to expand in order to accommodate a growing child and for childbirth. However, excessive progesterone has a downside: it also means that a pregnant woman is more prone to injury. Avoid jerky, bouncy, or high-impact motions to keep from hurting yourself.

Carrying extra pounds causes your body to work harder, even when you're doing the same amount of exercise to which you're accustomed. The additional weight in your front shifts your center of gravity, stressing the joints and the muscles in your lower back and pelvis.

As the second trimester comes to a close, you may have more back pain and become prone to losing your balance. You might feel more confident with exercise programs that are designed for pregnant women, including yoga and aerobics.

Your growing uterus will probably press on your diaphragm, making it harder to take the deep breaths you need when you're working out. If you're able to carry on a normal conversation during exercise, then you are within an acceptable range for exertion. Swimming or water aerobics will alleviate the pressure on your diaphragm.

Do not exercise while lying flat on your back now. Lying down compresses a large blood vessel called the *vena cava*. The vena cava shuttles blood to and from the heart, so pressing on it could cause a sudden drop in blood pressure, dizziness, or a loss of consciousness. Other changes in circulation caused by extra pounds slow blood flow, so fluid retention in your legs and ankles is more likely than before.

Although it's important to be careful when you're working out, don't let the caveats deter you from regular physical activity. You're doing yourself and your baby a big favor when you exercise on most days of the week. Being in shape before delivery usually means a faster return to fitness after giving birth.

> WORDS OF
> *Motherly Wisdom*
>
> "I'm in my second trimester now. I wear a heart-rate monitor when I work out because I've been told to keep my heart rate under 140 beats per minute."
> —*Kasie*

The Third Trimester (Weeks 27 to 40)

What's Going On in There?

You're in the home stretch. In just a short while, your baby will debut. A child is considered full-term at thirty-seven weeks, but the goal is forty.

Your child is really growing now. From the start of the third trimester to delivery day (about 13 weeks), the baby's body weight will double, and your weight gain will largely reflect that gain in heft as the baby adds fat and accumulates nutrients such as calcium and iron.

Third-Trimester To-Do List

WORDS OF
Motherly Wisdom

"With all three of my kids, I always found the last trimester to be both nerve-wracking and exciting. I couldn't wait to see my new baby!"
—*Shana*

- Discuss your birth plan with the doctor or midwife who will deliver your bundle of joy. Take a prenatal class to help ease delivery-day fears.
- Find a pediatrician. Check with your insurance company, get advice from friends, or ask your hospital for a referral.
- Get a group B strep culture. Some women carry strep B, a normally harmless bacteria that can cause infection in newborns. Women who test positive should receive antibiotics during labor.
- Buy a car seat and make sure it's properly installed. You won't be allowed to leave the hospital without one.
- Prepare to feed. If you're going to breast-feed, purchase a breast pump and learn how to use it now. Make sure you have a supply of comfortable clothes you can easily nurse in, as well as nursing bras and nursing pads. All parents should stock up on bottles and nipples. Even if you plan to breast-feed, you may eventually want to pump milk so that someone other than you can feed your child. If you're not planning to nurse, don't forget to buy infant formula.

The baby's organs, most notably the brain and the lungs, continue to mature to handle life outside the womb. Your baby's brain development is rapid from about the twenty-fourth week on, and the eyes are preparing to take in the world very soon. By birth, your child will probably measure nineteen to twenty-one inches from head to toe. Babies can either have a full head of hair or be completely bald when they arrive.

Whether you plan on nursing your child or not, your breasts are counting on it. You may have noticed a recent expansion as they prepare to produce milk.

Toward the end of your pregnancy, you should be checking in with your physician or midwife on a weekly basis (more often if you're having more than one baby) to monitor your health and your baby's health.

What to Eat Now

It's as important as ever to continue taking a daily multivitamin and other supplements, such as extra iron and calcium, as needed.

Your calorie needs in the third trimester are the highest they'll be during your entire pregnancy. The irony is that you need to eat more— 450 additional calories over prepregnancy needs—but as your due date approaches, you may find it more and more difficult to work in all those calories. Your expanding uterus and the baby it carries crowd your stomach in the third trimester. A cramped abdominal area is probably to blame for heartburn, too. Try dividing up your calorie allowance into six small, nourishing meals. Read more about handling heartburn in chapter 8.

Toward the end of the trimester, you might not be sleeping as well because it can be difficult to get comfortable. Healthy eating can't cure your fatigue, but it certainly can help. Eat more frequently to keep your energy level as high as possible. Another irritation will be pressure on your bladder, which means that you'll probably get up a few times at night to pee and will also need to go frequently during the day. Restricting fluid intake won't help, however. Try lying on your side to take the stress off your kidneys, and always empty your bladder before retiring for the night.

The third trimester is the time of extremely rapid brain growth. Your child's brain size increases by nearly 260 percent from about the twenty-fourth week of pregnancy to the fortieth. It's especially important to include the nutrients your child needs to support brain development, including protein, omega-3 fats such as DHA, and choline, which are discussed in detail in chapter 2.

Exercise During the Third Trimester: Keep Going

Your body is gearing up for delivery, so it's probably more limber than you think. It's especially important to pay attention to how you feel during exercise; avoid pushing yourself in order to avoid muscle strain.

By the end of the pregnancy, you probably won't be doing much more than walking, swimming, or prenatal exercise classes, because everything else might be too uncomfortable, given your size and the change in your center of gravity. Nevertheless, many women work out right up until delivery day. Just remember to take it at your own pace, and be sure to drink enough fluids.

Gestational Diabetes

Between the twenty-fourth and twenty-eighth weeks of your pregnancy, you should have a blood test for gestational diabetes mellitus (GDM). GDM is the form of diabetes that occurs for the first time when a woman is pregnant. See chapter 7 for the details about GDM.

Prepare Your Kitchen

You might not know whether you're having a boy or a girl, but one thing is for sure: you'll be busy after the baby is born, and you won't have time to prepare complicated meals. Eating properly after delivery is central to bouncing back from nine months of pregnancy and childbirth, however. It's especially important for nursing mothers. Avoid "flying by the seat of your pants" once the baby arrives. Stock your cupboards, refrigerator, and freezer with foods now to get you through the first few months with a minimum of fuss.

Load up on canned and frozen foods that are easy to prepare in a pinch, including fruits, vegetables, canned light tuna fish,

> WORDS OF
> *Motherly Wisdom*
>
> "I bought a separate freezer when I was pregnant and did a lot of food preparation so that I'd have something in reserve."
> —*Janice*

> WORDS OF
> *Motherly Wisdom*
>
> "I live in an area where a lot of the local take-out and delivery restaurants serve healthy cuisine, such as Japanese, Thai, and Middle Eastern, so I kept those menus close by during the months after my son was born."
> —*Dina*

salmon, and beans (chickpeas, black beans, and edamame). Purchase red meat, poultry, and seafood, such as bags of frozen shrimp, to freeze, labeling each package with the amount and the date you put it in the freezer. Make sure you have condiments on hand, including balsamic and red wine vinegars, olive and canola oils, jelly or jam, ketchup, mayonnaise, mustard, salad dressing, and any others that you enjoy. Purchase boxes of whole-grain cereal, pasta, whole grains (such as quick-cooking brown rice, wild rice, and whole-wheat couscous), and nut butters (peanut or almond) or sunflower seed butter. Add frozen whole-wheat pizza crusts to your kitchen survival grocery list.

Begin preparing meals, such as large batches of casseroles, lasagnas, stews, and soups, to freeze. If space is tight, consider buying a chest freezer. Label each gallon-size container or resealable storage bag (great because you can freeze them lying flat and they don't take up as much room, and you're not tying up all of your heavy-duty plastic containers) with the date of preparation.

Decision Time: How Will You Feed Your Baby?

You've decorated the baby's room and have even decided on a name for your impending arrival. Have you given much thought to how you'll feed your baby?

Breast milk is one of nature's most perfectly designed foods and, as such, is considered the best choice for newborns and infants. Several health organizations, including the American Academy of Pediatrics, recommend nursing a child for at least twelve months. Don't let that time frame scare you; any amount of nursing is beneficial to your baby and to you.

Perhaps you have been unsuccessful at nursing in the past. This doesn't mean that you'll have trouble with this baby. If you have other children and you've never nursed before, give it a try. You can always start with nursing your baby and switch to infant formula, but, in general, you can't start with formula and switch to breast-feeding—at least,

> WORDS OF
> *Motherly Wisdom*
>
> "I was nervous about nursing because my mother never did, and a lot of friends had no experience with it, so I didn't know whom I could turn to for advice. Still, I tried it, and it worked out great for me and my children."
> —*Shana*

not after the first few days after delivery have passed (although it's not impossible).

At this point, you might be adamant about formula feeding. You're just not interested in being the sole source of nutrition for your child, or maybe you're going back to work in a few months and you think that breast-feeding is out of the question. There's no need to fret about mixing breast-feeding with a return to work, however. There are many ways to make nursing work when you are away from your baby for hours at a time, such as pumping breast milk that your baby takes from a bottle from someone else. Even if you nurse your child for a short time before returning to work, then switch the feedings to infant formula, you will still have done your baby a world of good.

Breast-Feeding: What's in It for You and Your Child

Breast milk is easily digested, and it contains all of the nutrients a baby needs for the first six months of life. Babies who nurse benefit in numerous ways from breast milk's protective qualities. Nursing infants tend to have fewer ear infections and diarrhea and less colic. Studies also suggest that breast-fed babies may be less likely to die from sudden infant death syndrome.

The health benefits of breast-feeding can last for your child's lifetime. Children and adults who were breast-fed as babies are less prone to asthma and allergies; insulin-dependent diabetes; and certain cancers, including leukemia, lymphoma, and Hodgkin's disease. Breast-fed babies are less likely to become overweight later in life, too.

Breast milk contains the healthy fats DHA and arachidonic acid (AA), which appear to promote brain development and possibly increase intelligence. Some studies found that children who were breast-fed scored higher on tests of cognitive ability than children who were fed formula. There is a caveat, however: the mother must consume adequate amounts of dietary DHA and AA in order to transfer it to her child through breast milk. See chapter 3 for more on these and other essential fats.

If breast milk has a fault, it is that it's low in vitamin D. The American Academy of Pediatrics recommends that all babies, including those who are exclusively breast-fed, consume at least 400 IU of vitamin D every day from the first days of life to help prevent rickets, a bone-weakening disease.

Besides being economical and convenient, breast-feeding is an amazing and rewarding experience for a woman and her child. Nursing aids in your body's ability to return to its prepregnancy state faster. Breast-feeding triggers the production of hormones that cause your uterus to contract, making it smaller and firmer. Nursing a child might also lower your risk of premenopausal breast cancer, ovarian cancer, and osteoporosis.

Nervous about Nursing?

You may be wondering if you'll be able to breast-feed successfully. It's normal to be nervous about nursing, especially with your first child, if you're having more than one baby at a time, or if you expect to deliver your baby before thirty-seven weeks. Speak with friends and family who have been successful at nursing or talk with your midwife, obstetrician, nurse practitioner, or a lactation consultant. Take a breast-feeding class at a local hospital to learn breast-feeding basics.

Who Should Not Breast-Feed?

Breast-feeding is recommended for nearly all mothers and their children, including mothers of multiple babies. However, there are some women who should not nurse, including the following:

- Women with HIV (human immunodeficiency virus, the virus that causes AIDS), because they can pass the virus on to their babies in their breast milk
- Women with active tuberculosis and who have not been treated with medications
- Women who are taking drugs for cancer treatment, including radio-active compounds
- Women who use illicit (recreational) drugs
- Women whose babies have galactosemia, a rare genetic disorder that impedes a baby's ability to process the carbohydrates in breast milk (and dairy-based formula). Newborn screening tests detect most babies with galactosemia soon after birth.

Women who have chronic health conditions that are controlled with medication (including prescription drugs, over-the-counter drugs, and herbal supplements) must check with their doctors before breast-feeding. Some medications and dietary supplements pose a risk to breast-feeding babies.

Women who have had breast surgery, such as breast enlargement or reduction, may be able to breast-feed, although some might have problems, such as not being able to produce enough milk.

Formula Feeding

Women choose formula for a number of reasons, including physical or medical reasons or because they plan on returning to work soon after delivering and don't think it will be convenient to pump milk or breast-feed at the office. Other mothers want to share the feeding responsibility, and they think that formula-feeding makes the best sense for all involved.

The makers of infant formula strive to come as close as possible to duplicating the composition of human milk, and they do an excellent job. Once you've decided on infant formula, the question becomes which one. Formulas based on cow's milk are a fine choice for most babies, unless they have an intolerance or a milk allergy. Make sure the formula you pick is fortified with iron so that your baby receives the right amount of this vital nutrient. Choose a formula that is also fortified with DHA and AA. In September 2007, the American Dietetic Association and the Dietitians of Canada published a joint position paper on dietary fatty acids. It stated that if you choose a human milk substitute (that is, infant formula) to feed your baby, the DHA level should be at least 0.2 percent of the total fatty acids, and the level of AA should not be lower than that of DHA. If the levels of DHA and AA are not listed on the infant formula label, contact the manufacturer to find out.

The next decision is the form of the formula. Infant formula comes as ready-to-feed, as concentrated liquid, or as powder. Powdered formulas are generally the least expensive, but they also require the most work to prepare. Nursing mothers who supplement their milk supply with powdered infant formula (such as those who travel out of town for work or those who are undergoing medical treatment) can conveniently mix up as much or as little formula as they need from powder, without waste. See chapter 5 for more on infant formula.

A Look at What's Ahead

In this chapter we explained the healthy lifestyle habits that will serve you well throughout each stage of pregnancy and that are beneficial after you deliver and even after you and your child are done with nursing. There's no need to stop taking such good care of yourself. Keep at it, especially if you're thinking about having more children.

The next chapter helps you to navigate the "fourth trimester," the period in which your body makes its way back to a nonpregnant state.

5

The Fourth Trimester: After the Baby Arrives

Congratulations on your new arrival! For the last nine months, and possibly longer, you've worked hard caring for yourself and your developing child. Now that delivery day has come and gone, you're on to the next phase of parenthood: the postpartum (after pregnancy) months, often referred to as the "fourth trimester."

During the fourth trimester, your body returns to its nonpregnant state. This early postpartum period is also when you and your family begin adjusting to life with a newborn, as you juggle new responsibilities and establish routines that work for you.

What's Happening Now

You were transformed during pregnancy, seemingly stretched to the limit as your due date approached. Furthermore, a long, arduous delivery may have left you worn out. After all, they don't call it labor for nothing! The chances are that you're sore, achy, and very tired.

If you had a cesarean delivery, you're recovering from the additional stress of surgery. You may have also some swelling that has yet to disappear. Postdelivery puffiness is even more likely with C-sections because of the intravenous fluids you received during the procedure. Don't worry; in a few days, you should start to lose the extra fluid you're carrying. Significant swelling, however, can signal a serious problem, such as a blood clot. If you're excessively puffy and have pain or swelling that's worse on one side of the body, let your health-care provider know immediately.

Swollen breasts are par for the course, beginning about two to five days after delivery. That's when milk production begins in earnest. Mothers who have decided to use infant formula can use cold compresses on their breasts to limit, and eventually prevent, milk production. For nursing women, breast engorgement is avoidable by nursing as often as your child wants to eat and by expressing extra milk with a breast pump when you're separated from your baby for long periods. Breast milk can be frozen or refrigerated for future use.

Expect some vaginal bleeding for up to six weeks after delivery. This is a normal occurrence, because the body is ridding itself of useless uterine tissue. Although mild bleeding during this time is considered normal, a fever and pain in the abdominal area are not. You may feel somewhat crampy at times, however, as your uterus shrinks back to its normal size; this is a process that can take months to complete.

You might experience constipation in the days just after delivery, especially if you received narcotics to ease labor pain, because they often slow down the digestive process. Hemorrhoids that developed from forceful pushing during delivery could also be plaguing you right now. See chapter 7 for how to relieve constipation and hemorrhoids.

Body (and Mind) After Baby

As you probably have discovered, taking care of your new little one is challenging and rewarding. You are no doubt giving your role 110 percent of your energy. However, don't neglect your own health in the name of motherhood. Ignoring your well-being for the sake of your baby will surely backfire. You may have less time right now to devote to eating right, relaxing, and regular physical activity, but caring for your body and your mind is as important as ever, especially if you're breast-feeding.

It can take months to regain your strength after the strain of pregnancy and childbirth, and it will probably take longer if you were on bed rest for weeks or months before the delivery, if you delivered your child by cesarean section, or if you had a complicated pregnancy.

Forget about trying to be Superwoman. Put the preparation of complicated meals for you and your family on the back burner, at least for a few months. Housework should not be your primary concern now, either. As for your career, or if you own a business, you may not get a lot of time off and need to go back to work fairly soon after delivering. No matter what situation you're in, the fourth trimester is not the time to try to do it all; delegating and seeking help is definitely what you should be doing now. There's no way that you can keep up the way you did before the baby was born without sacrificing much-needed energy, so it's pointless to try. Instead, nap when the baby naps. Don't use that precious time to pay the bills, clean the bathroom, or do the laundry. There's plenty of time for chores later.

You need support, so don't feel bad asking for it. Allow others to help you out as much as possible, even if it's simply to watch your baby while you do a few quick errands, take a nap, or enjoy a meal. Hire a cleaning service, if you are able to afford it, or work out a plan to share the responsibility with your spouse or partner and other family members. Create your own informal mothers' support group or join one in your community. Always accept donations of food. It's wonderful to know you have something nourishing to eat on hand after a tiring day with your infant.

The early months of motherhood are taxing. Take time each day to enjoy your newborn—who will grow very quickly. Nevertheless, don't forget about you. Set aside a half hour or so each day to shower or take a bath, to relax with a book or listen to music, or to get some fresh air.

Postpartum Appointments

If the postpartum period is problem-free for you, the next visit you'll have with your doctor or other appropriate licensed health-care professional should come four to six weeks after delivery—probably sooner if you had a cesarean delivery or a complicated pregnancy.

WORDS OF
Motherly Wisdom

"Never, ever say no to an offer of help. The first few weeks after birth is no time to be a hero."
—*Lisa*

The appointment should include a thorough physical exam. Use the visit to discuss any aspect of your health, including how you're adjusting emotionally to your role as a parent; how the new baby is affecting your relationship with your spouse or partner; your fatigue level; when you can start exercising again and how much you can do; and any other issue that pertains to your well-being.

Identifying Postpartum Depression

Do you cry for no discernable reason? Maybe you lash out at your loved ones even when they are trying to be helpful. Perhaps you're harboring intense feelings of anger and resentment as you get up to feed your child for the third time during the night while your husband sleeps soundly. If so, you're not alone.

Like nearly all mothers, you find it challenging to live up to the increased demands on your limited time and flagging energy. The "baby blues," which include mood swings, weepiness, an inability to concentrate, and anxiety, can last for days or several weeks. The exact causes are unclear, but rapid changes in hormone levels, the physical and emotional stress of giving birth, sleep deprivation, and disappointment about life after the baby is born are some of the reasons the experts cite. However, even though you may be concerned about these postpartum emotions, the chances are that they'll pass.

Problems arise when you can't shake the sadness. If you feel anxious, hopeless, or constantly irritable; if you have trouble sleeping; if you feel little connection between you and your newborn; or if you fear harming yourself or your child, you may have postpartum depression, a serious medical condition that can develop any time during the first year after delivery. Women who experienced depression during pregnancy or after a previous pregnancy are particularly prone to postpartum depression.

It's important that you receive treatment for the way you feel. When a mother is depressed, for any reason, every member of the family, particularly infants and young children, are affected. For example, depressed mothers spend less time looking at, talking to, and touching their babies, activities that foster brain development and inspire feelings of trust in the child. Depressed mothers are also less likely to be sensitive to the child's emotional needs.

What You Should Eat Now

Mothers with newborn babies constantly battle exhaustion. A healthy lifestyle is no substitute for a good night's sleep, but eating right and getting regular physical activity do lessen fatigue and stress. Nutritious food provides you with the energy to cope with a needy infant who seems to eat all day long, to cry for no reason for hours at a time, and to require a dozen or more diaper changes a day. In addition to this, perhaps you are also managing other children, a household, and a career. A balanced eating plan will help your body to heal.

To make your recovery go smoothly, finish taking the remainder of your prenatal vitamins, along with other supplements, such as calcium, if necessary. When your prenatal vitamins run out, substitute a daily multivitamin that provides close to 100 percent of the Daily Value of the nutrients it contains, including iron and folic acid. There's no need for a supplement that provides more, in spite of the promotion of this for nursing mothers.

After a few weeks, or maybe a month, you'll probably start yearning to fit into your prepregnancy clothes. Nevertheless, hold off on trying to squeeze into your jeans for at least six weeks after delivery to allow your body to mend. Follow a balanced eating plan with a minimum of 1,800 calories (nursing mothers may need more calories; see page 134) to allow your body to recover from nine months of pregnancy and the act of childbirth. Rely on a MyPyramid plan to guide you to safe weight loss. Do not skip meals, especially breakfast.

Even though there's no rush, make sure you try to shed pregnancy pounds during the first year after delivery by getting some physical activity on most days of the week and by following a MyPyramid plan that provides the right number of calories for weight loss. (See chapter 3 for more information on healthy eating plans to help with weight loss.) Research suggests that it's harder to take off pregnancy weight after twelve months have passed.

> ### WORDS OF
> ### *Motherly Wisdom*
>
> "The night after coming home from the hospital with my first baby, I was so excited to have my favorite broccoli and onion pizza, because most of what I had read said that my diet wouldn't affect my baby. What a mistake! Neither one of us slept the entire night. His stomach was so upset!"
> —*Kasie*

Special Considerations for Nursing Mothers

As a nursing mother, you need about the same number of extra calories you did during the second trimester: 330 a day. If you nurse past six months, increase your daily intake by about 400 calories more than your prepregnancy needs, or about the amount you consumed in the third trimester. You need more protein when nursing than during pregnancy. Nursing women require 0.59 grams of protein per pound of body weight plus an additional 25 grams every day. That amounts to about 105 grams of protein a day for a 135-pound woman. When you follow the MyPyramid Postpregnancy Plan with adequate calories for your physical activity level and take a daily multivitamin, it's unlikely that you or your baby will lack any nutrient, with the possible exception of DHA.

Breast-feeding women need 200 to 300 mg of DHA every day to help maximize the baby's brain and visual development. Getting enough omega-3 fats, particularly DHA, can be problematic if you don't include fish or foods fortified with DHA, such as eggs (see chapter 2 for more on DHA). You will need a supplement if your diet does not provide enough of this important fat.

Although breast milk is considered the perfect food for babies, it lacks adequate vitamin D to protect their growing bones. Vitamin D is essential to the movement of calcium in and out of the bones, and it's particularly powerful for preventing rickets, which causes soft, weak bones in children. Vitamin D production starts in skin that's been exposed to strong sunlight and finishes in the liver and kidneys. Technically, your child's body can make all of the vitamin D it needs. However, it's unlikely that your infant will produce adequate vitamin D, because most babies don't spend enough time in the sunlight to provoke vitamin D production. That's why the American Academy of Pediatrics recommends 400 international units (IU) of supplemental vitamin D every day for breast-fed infants, beginning in the first days of life. (Infant formula contains adequate vitamin D.) If you are nursing, your pediatrician should prescribe a vitamin D supplement for your child.

Now that you're finished with pregnancy, you'd probably like to go back to having a glass of wine with dinner or a martini or two when you're out. Not so fast—an occasional drink is probably okay when you're nursing, but it's not advisable to make it a habit. Alcohol gets into breast milk. It can slow the development of your child's motor skills, which influences activities like walking and grabbing large objects. Beer, wine, and hard liquor can also interfere with your baby's ability to get milk from you during nursing. Alcohol inhibits the production of oxytocin, a hormone that encourages the flow of breast milk. If you do try nursing while alcohol is active in your system, don't be surprised if you have difficulty "letting down"—getting the milk to flow easily.

You may also be eager to smoke cigarettes again now that you're no longer pregnant, but it's not a good idea. Nicotine and other harmful chemicals in cigarettes make their way into your milk supply. Moreover, smoking around a newborn raises the risk of sudden infant death syndrome. Secondhand smoke is dangerous for newborns, young children, and everyone else, so if you quit smoking while you were pregnant, it really doesn't make any sense to start again.

Try not to rely too heavily on caffeine for an energy boost. Caffeine may provide the jolt you need to keep going as the mother of a newborn, but keep in mind that it will have the same effect on your child, maybe even more so. Babies don't process caffeine as quickly as adults, so consuming it can leave you with a child who is irritable and has difficulty settling down to go to sleep, perhaps just when you're completely worn out and looking forward to some rest. For your sake and the baby's, limit coffee, tea, and other caffeine-containing beverages, and foods, when you're nursing to well under 200 mg a day (see chapter 2 for more on caffeine).

Focus on Fluoride

Although the water supplies in most U.S. cities and towns are bolstered by fluoride—a chemical that can help teeth and nails to grow strong—the levels can be low in certain areas. Ask your local water company how many parts per million of fluoride is in your drinking water. If the level is below 3 parts per million, consult your pediatrician about whether your baby should take fluoride supplements. The American Dental Association and the American Academy of Pediatrics advise that fluoride supplementation begin at six months for breast-fed and formula-fed infants.

Making a Meal in Ten Minutes or Less

You're a busy new mother with little time to feed yourself. These meals might not be your idea of gourmet, but they do the trick in a pinch, and they fit perfectly into any MyPyramid eating plan.

- 1 hard-cooked egg, 8 ounces low-fat yogurt, 1 slice whole-grain toast, and fruit.
- Stuffed baked potato: Microwave a medium white potato or use a leftover cooked potato. Scoop out the inside and mix with 1 cup low-fat, low-sodium cottage cheese. Return the filling to the potato skin. Add a green salad.
- 1-ounce whole-wheat bagel with 2 tablespoons peanut butter, almond butter, or sunflower seed butter. Serve with 8 ounces 1% low-fat milk.
- Pita pizza: Broil 1 small whole-wheat pita round covered with tomato sauce and 1 ounce reduced-fat grated cheese until the cheese has melted. Serve with 8 ounces 100% orange juice.
- Sunflower seed butter and raisin or banana sandwich on whole-grain bread: 2 slices whole-grain bread, 2 tablespoons sunflower seed butter, and 1 small banana, sliced, or 2 tablespoons raisins.
- Quick quesadilla: Place one 7-inch whole-wheat sandwich wrap in a medium skillet coated with nonstick cooking spray and layer with 2 ounces chopped, cooked chicken and 1 ounce reduced-fat cheddar cheese. Cover with another 7-inch whole-wheat sandwich wrap and heat until the cheese has melted. Serve with a piece of fruit.
- Egg in a pocket: Scramble an egg or two and place in half of a whole-wheat pita pocket. Top with salsa and 1 ounce reduced-fat cheese, if desired. Serve with an 8-ounce glass of low-fat 1% milk.
- 3 ounces salmon, fresh or canned, 1 cup cooked whole-grain couscous, and 1 cup frozen vegetables, cooked.
- 1 egg, scrambled, with ¼ cup grated reduced-fat cheddar cheese, 1 slice whole-wheat toast and jam. Serve with 8 ounces fortified 100% orange juice.
- 3 ounces canned light tuna, 10 whole-grain crackers, and a piece of fruit.
- Stuffed melon: Slice a honeydew or cantaloupe melon in half. Scoop out the seeds. Place 1 cup low-fat, low-sodium cottage cheese or low-fat vanilla or plain yogurt in the hollow section. Serve with a 1-ounce whole-wheat roll.
- 1 cup canned reduced-sodium lentil soup mixed with 1 cup cooked pasta. Serve with 8 ounces 1% low-fat milk and a piece of fruit.
- Combine 1 cup canned white beans, drained, with 1 tablespoon olive oil and 3 ounces shrimp in a skillet. Cook until the shrimp are pink. Serve with a piece of fruit.

- Stir-fry ½ pound ground turkey or lean ground beef with chopped onions and cumin. Spoon the cooked meat onto whole-wheat tortillas along with chopped tomato, lettuce, and low-fat sour cream. (This dish serves two.) Serve with a piece of fruit.
- Coat 4 ounces thinly sliced chicken breasts or tenders with flour. Heat 1 tablespoon olive oil in a medium skillet. Cook chicken for about two minutes on each side. Pile onto a whole-wheat sandwich bun and garnish with tomato and lettuce. Serve with 8 ounces 1% low-fat milk and a piece of fruit.
- Quick fried rice: Heat 2 teaspoons canola oil in a medium skillet. Add 1 cup cold cooked white or brown rice, ¼ cup chopped onion, ¼ cup cooked peas or diced carrots or both, and 1 beaten egg. Toss the entire mixture until the egg is cooked. Season with a dash of low-sodium soy sauce. Serve with a piece of fruit.
- Put 4 ounces cooked shrimp or light canned tuna, drained, on 2 cups leafy greens and ½ cup grape tomatoes and top with 2 teaspoons olive oil and balsamic vinegar. Serve with 1 slice (1 ounce) whole-grain bread and 8 ounces low-sodium vegetable juice.

Dodging Deficiency: Vitamin B$_{12}$

If you shun all animal foods, you and your baby could be at risk for a deficiency in vitamin B$_{12}$, which is found naturally only in animal foods. It's especially important for you to take a daily multivitamin with at least 100 percent of the Daily Value of vitamin B$_{12}$, whether you're nursing or not. Include fortified foods such as breakfast cereals, soy and other plant-based beverages, nutrition bars, meat substitutes, and fortified brewer's yeast in your eating plan, too.

Breast-Feeding Basics

Your child is ready to breast-feed just moments after birth. That will be obvious to you when you see how instinctively your baby roots for your breast while being held close. It may therefore seem ironic that your milk doesn't come in until a few days after delivery. During the initial days after delivery, your baby gets colostrum, or "first milk," from you, which is clear or yellow fluid. Colostrum provides what your child needs just after birth, including antibodies, which are disease-fighting compounds.

Your breasts will swell as your milk comes in. Frequent breast-feeding is important because it builds up your milk supply. Nurse as often as your baby wants to eat; it's good for your child and alleviates breast discomfort for you, too. You'll know when it's time to nurse by your baby's wide-open eyes and sucking motions. Nurse before fussiness or hunger sets in; otherwise it will be difficult for your baby to calm down and eat. Allow somewhat sleepy babies to wake up a bit first before feeding.

Breast-feeding a baby is a natural bodily function, but it doesn't always come naturally to a woman, especially one who has never nursed before, who has had a difficult labor and delivery, or both. You may have received excellent instructions about nursing your baby and received wonderful support from the staff at the hospital, but now that you're on your own, you may be thinking twice about this breast-feeding business. You are not alone; it's very normal for nursing mothers, particularly first-timers, to feel overwhelmed during the first two or three weeks after delivery and even longer.

WORDS OF
Motherly Wisdom

"Nobody talks about how painful nursing can be during the first few weeks. Still, it's well worth it."
—*Teri*

Giving up on nursing is especially attractive when you're having any pain or discomfort associated with breast-feeding. Get help instead. Even when you don't have friends or family who are knowledgeable about breast-feeding, there are plenty of others, including certified lactation consultants, who are willing to help you learn to nurse your child. Lactation consultants, who work in hospitals and other health-care settings, often make house calls and can help you work through the rough spots you have at any time. Lactation consultants are knowledgeable about a variety of issues, including feeding a preterm baby and combining a return to work with breast-feeding. An International Board Certified Lactation Consultant is a health-care professional, such as a nurse or a registered dietitian, who is certified by the International Board of Lactation Consultant Examiners. Visit the International Lactation Consultant Association's Web site, www.ilca.org, to find a certified lactation consultant in your area.

Sleep deprivation, too, can prompt thoughts of giving up on breast-feeding. It may be of some comfort to know that newborns generally do not sleep through the night for the first few months. Switching to infant formula will not help your baby to sleep longer. In fact, whether bottle-fed or breast-fed, newborns should eat about eight to twelve times a day. They really should not go any longer than four hours without eating during the first three or four weeks, which thus entails nighttime feedings.

Nothing but the Breast

The American Academy of Pediatrics recommends only breast milk for breast-fed babies for about the first six months of life. There is no need to give your baby water or any other liquids or solids, although it's fine to start solid foods between four and six months of age, depending on your baby's readiness. The goal is to continue nursing after solid foods are introduced and for at least twelve months. Continue breast-feeding after your baby turns one year old for as long as you and your child desire.

Infant Formula Preparation

Always follow the manufacturer's directions for formula preparation. That might seem obvious to you, but parents don't always heed the advice. A study in the *Journal of the American Dietetic Association* found that one-third of the mothers who were surveyed used warm water directly from the tap to mix infant formula even though the recommendation is to use tap water that has been boiled and cooled. The water (tap or bottled) that is used to prepare concentrated and powdered infant formula must be boiled for at least five minutes to reduce the risk of bacterial contamination that could sicken the baby. In the same study, nearly half of the mothers heated baby bottles in a microwave oven, a practice that's discouraged because of the risk of burns to a baby's mouth.

There's a good chance that the tap water in your home contains added fluoride, which is important to young children's tooth development, particularly before their primary teeth start showing through their gums. (Boiling tap water does not affect water's fluoride level.) Most bottled water, which you may choose to use to prepare infant formula, does not provide fluoride, however. If you prefer bottled water instead of tap, make sure it contains fluoride. Call the bottled water company to find out the fluoride content and ask your pediatrician if that level is sufficient.

Your house, apartment, or condominium might have lead pipes that leach lead into your drinking water, particularly if the building was constructed prior to 1988. More recent dwellings are not necessarily safe, because copper pipes can be connected with lead solder that gets into tap water, too. Make sure your water supply is lead-free before you use it for infant formula. (See chapter 6 for more on lead.)

Is Your Baby Eating Enough?

Babies are great self-regulators—they know when they are full, so they should be allowed to eat as much or as little as they desire. A breast-fed baby who is satisfied will release the nipple and turn away from the breast. Never force a child to eat, but do encourage your baby to nurse long enough to soften at least one breast during every feeding (start with the other breast for the next feeding). The richer, fattier milk becomes available at the end of the feeding.

Nursing newborns should eat eight to twelve times a day during the first month. If your child has at least six wet diapers every twenty-four hours and three bowel movements a day by the end of the first week of life and is steadily gaining weight, that should be fine. Ask your pediatrician, if you have doubts. The doctor will probably want to check your child three to five days after birth to determine if your child is gaining an adequate amount of weight.

Babies typically experience growth spurts, so be prepared for eating to increase between eight and twelve days old, at about three to four weeks old, and at three months old. Spurts vary thereafter through the first year of life.

Your Colicky Child

Newborns fuss; it's the way they let you know that they need something. However, screaming fits that start suddenly on a daily basis, usually in late afternoon or evening, and last for more than about three hours are another matter. Your child may have colic.

An estimated one in five babies has colic, which typically shows up at about three weeks and peaks by six weeks of age; then it starts to wane, albeit slowly. No matter what the duration, colic is stressful and frustrating for parents.

The cause of colic is a mystery. A colicky child could be hypersensitive to stimulation or uncomfortable because of intestinal gas. Before labeling your child colicky, check with your pediatrician to be sure your child's distress is not due to a medical problem, such as a hernia or an infection. If your child is still wailing on a daily basis by three months of age, it might be due to a condition called reflux, in which the stomach contents flow backward into the esophagus, causing a burning sensation.

Call your doctor immediately if your baby's behavior or crying pattern changes suddenly or if your crying child has a fever, forceful vomiting, diarrhea, bloody stools, or anything else out of the ordinary.

Diet can make a difference in children with colic. Hungry babies may cry incessantly; overfed children may, too. For example, if bottle feedings take less than twenty minutes, the hole in the nipple could be too large, leading to a bellyache for the baby. Nursing children with colic might not tolerate certain foods in their mothers' diets. Maybe you've heard that nursing mothers should avoid gas-producing foods such as broccoli, cabbage, and legumes. Although there's not much evidence that this alleviates colic in a breast-fed baby, if you find that these, or any other foods, are particularly irritating, leave them out of your diet for the time being. If you eliminate an entire food group, you will need advice from a registered dietitian on how to make up for the nutrients you are missing. Avoid caffeine to limit stimulation in your child.

Certain proteins in infant formula can irritate a baby's intestinal tract. Some children respond well to a formula change, but discuss any alterations in feeding with your pediatrician first. In general, colicky infants are as likely as infants without colic to eat well and gain weight normally.

Figuring out what to do to comfort your child and how to reduce the stress you feel as a parent during this rocky time is critical for managing colic. Holding your child as much as possible, even when the baby is not fussy, could prevent colic later in the day. Gentle rocking and being held upright can also help to relieve your child's intestinal distress.

When to Start Exercising After Birth

You just had a baby, and it seems as if you're in constant motion as you try to run the household, work, and take care of yourself and your family. That's why you probably don't need to exercise as you did before—at least not within the first few months after delivery.

In fact, pushing yourself too hard too early after delivery is counterproductive, because it saps the energy required to take care of your new baby. It can even be dangerous, if you lost a lot of blood during childbirth, had a cesarean delivery, delivered more than one baby, or were on bed rest for weeks or months before the delivery.

If everything went well during pregnancy and delivery, most women can begin walking for exercise a few weeks after having a child; others will need to wait longer. Typically, women get approval for working out at their six-week checkup. Discuss your situation with your health-care provider. Once your doctor, nurse practitioner, or nurse-midwife gives you the go-ahead, a gradual return to your prepregnancy level of physical activity is the best strategy.

If you had a cesarean section, you know that you've undergone major abdominal surgery. Like all women, you will be encouraged to return to exercise as soon as it is safe to do so. However, having a C-section means that this will take longer. Women who have had cesarean deliveries are advised to avoid climbing stairs or lifting heavy objects until the incision has healed. Walking only very short distances at first is the best path to recovery. Don't do anything that causes pain or discomfort at the incision site. There's no point in rushing to exercise. Ask your health-care provider what's right for you.

Even if you want to work out, you might wonder if it's worth spending what little free time you have on aerobics, yoga, or Pilates. You may prefer to get exercise that allows you to include your baby. Take a walk with the baby in the carrier or the stroller. When the weather is bad, use an exercise videotape or DVD at home and bounce around the room while your baby watches.

Exercise can help you to lose weight as long as you're eating the right number of calories to shed pounds. A combination of calorie reduction and regular physical activity helps you to drop the pounds while preserving muscle tissue. The latter is important, since muscle burns more calories overall than fat does. You need to exercise even if weight loss is not your goal, however. Physical activity is important for women of all ages because it helps to prevent pounds from creeping up on you as you age; it also builds and tones muscles, increases stamina and cardiovascular fitness, and enhances mental health.

Breast-feeding mothers should try to nurse just before exercising for prolonged periods (thirty minutes or more) to avoid discomfort and to avoid any potential problems with acidity. Breast milk becomes more acidic from lactic acid, a compound that is produced by working muscles. The acidity is not usually a problem, but some infants might not like the taste. Drink fluids before, during, and after exercise to stay hydrated. Wear a comfortable bra that provides the support you need when you're working out.

Ideas for Short Exercise Sessions

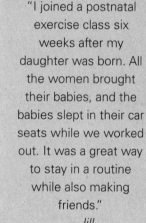

WORDS OF
Motherly Wisdom

"I joined a postnatal exercise class six weeks after my daughter was born. All the women brought their babies, and the babies slept in their car seats while we worked out. It was a great way to stay in a routine while also making friends."
—*Jill*

It's not always easy to work in thirty continuous minutes of physical activity, but most mothers have time for at least ten minutes a day. Start off with a ten-minute block of activity daily and work your way up to at least three. You can string them together or mix and match. For example, take a brisk thirty-minute walk or ride a bike for twenty minutes and do resistance training for ten. Following are some activities that fit nicely in ten-minute blocks:

- A brisk walk (defined as a fifteen-minute mile) at the mall, during a coffee break or a lunch break, on a treadmill, or while pushing your child in a stroller
- A slow jog
- Bicycle riding (ten miles per hour)
- Resistance training. Repeat this sequence for ten minutes: ten sit-ups, ten push-ups, ten biceps curls with light weights, ten squats, and ten jumping jacks
- Swimming
- Use of an elliptical machine
- Use of a stair-stepping machine
- Dancing

- Low-impact aerobics
- Yoga
- Water aerobics

Simple Ways to Burn Off Calories

Fool yourself into exercise with these everyday activities that burn about 100 calories for a 150-pound person. If you weigh more, you'll burn more. If you weigh less, you'll burn less, so it will take longer to work off 100 calories.

Do This	For This Many Minutes
Run up the stairs throughout the day	6
Walk up the stairs throughout the day	11
Run in place	11
Kick a soccer ball around with your children	13
Shovel snow	15
Play hopscotch	18
Shoot hoops	20
Mow the lawn	20
Play golf (no cart)	20
Do light yard work	20
Play tag with your children	22
Fly a kite	22
Ride a bike (about ten miles per hour)	22
Toss a Frisbee	29
Carry a small child	29
Wash the car	30
Bowl	30
Throw a ball with your children	30
Explore the zoo while pushing a child in a stroller	35
Sit and play with your toddler	35
Stretch gently	35
Type on a computer	50

Adapted from Ainsworth, B. et al. "Compendium of Physical Activities: An Update of Activity Codes and MET Intensities." Medicine & Science in Sports and Exercise, 32(9 Suppl): S498–504, 2000.

Work Out Together

Parenthood can be a lonely endeavor; so can working out and eating right. Make your life easier by joining a mother-and-baby stroller-walking and fitness group, such as Stroller Strides or StrollerFit, or find another new mother or two to walk with or to swap babysitting with while you work out.

Preparing for Your Next Pregnancy

You love your new little one so deeply that perhaps you're already thinking about having another. However, even though it's never too early for women and their partners to prepare for pregnancy, you should probably wait at least a year before trying to conceive.

Having two babies in quick succession can jeopardize the well-being of the second one, according to a recent study in the *Journal of the American Medical Association*. The study suggests that a gap of eighteen months to just under five years is ideal. The researchers found that infants born outside that time frame were significantly more likely to be preterm and have a low birth weight.

Whether you should do anything differently from what you did to prepare yourself for the next baby depends on the type of pregnancy you had. If you developed complications when you were pregnant, such as iron deficiency or excessive weight gain, be prepared to consider them when you are ready to conceive again. It is possible to conceive when you're nursing, so take precautions if you don't want to become pregnant just yet.

Habits for Life

Once the fourth trimester ends or you stop nursing, you might be tempted to revert to your not-so-healthy ways, but try hard not to do so. Pregnancy and the postpartum period probably motivated you more than ever to eat right, exercise, and get the rest you need. Maintain your healthy habits as time passes. You have a family now, so eating right and exercising will serve you well, especially if you plan to add to your family in the coming years.

6

Food Safety: Before, During, and After Pregnancy

I t's always important to be mindful of food safety, but it's even more critical just before and during pregnancy. Pregnant women run a greater risk for food-borne illness (sickness caused by eating tainted food) because of a weakened immune system that makes it harder for the body to fend off germs.

When you're expecting, or planning on it, you want to protect your child and yourself as much as possible. Food safety is mostly in your hands. Armed with some basic knowledge, mothers-to-be can ward off exposure to germs and other potentially harmful contaminants.

Problematic Bacteria and Other Germs

Food has all of the qualities that germs desire: a source of nutrition, water, and warmth. Since no food is considered completely sterile, it's important to handle and store food properly. Bacteria, viruses, and parasites all cause food-borne illness, but bacteria are responsible for most sickness. Here are some of the most dangerous conditions caused by germs.

Listeriosis

Listeriosis is caused by *Listeria monocytogenes* (or *Listeria*), a harmful bacterium with serious consequences for a mother and her unborn child. You're twenty times more likely to get listeriosis when you're expecting, mostly because your resistance to germs is lower then. About one-third of listeriosis cases occur in pregnant women, and the condition can be passed to your baby.

Listeriosis is troublesome. During the first trimester of pregnancy, it is capable of causing miscarriage. It can also result in preterm delivery, low-birth-weight babies, and infant death. In newborns, listeriosis causes blood infections and meningitis.

Most of the time, pregnant women with listeriosis don't feel sick. When listeriosis does produce symptoms—such as fever, chills, muscle aches, diarrhea or upset stomach, headache, stiff neck, confusion, and loss of balance—it can be mistaken for something else. Because listeriosis is often elusive, it's important to do everything possible to prevent it.

Among bacteria, *Listeria* is unusual because it's capable of growing at refrigerator temperatures (about 40°F), whereas most other food-borne bacteria cannot. *Listeria* is capable of contaminating refrigerated, ready-to-eat meat and seafood, unpasteurized dairy products and foods made with them, and even soil. You can also get listeriosis by consuming foods that have been processed or packaged in unsanitary conditions or by eating vegetables that are contaminated from the soil or from manure used as fertilizer.

Listeriosis can generally be thwarted with a few easy strategies. (See "Simple Steps to Safer Food" later in this chapter for more tips.) Stay away from the following foods:

- Hot dogs and luncheon meats, such as ham, turkey, and bologna, unless they're reheated until steaming hot.
- Soft cheeses such as feta, Brie, Camembert, blue-veined cheese, *queso blanco, queso fresco,* and Panela—*unless* they're made with pasteurized milk. Check the label to be certain.
- Refrigerated pâtés or meat spreads.

- Refrigerated smoked seafood, including smoked salmon, trout, whitefish, cod, tuna, and mackerel. These products may be labeled *nova-style, lox, kippered, smoked,* or *jerky.* They are typically offered in the refrigerator section or sold at deli counters of grocery stores and delicatessens. It's fine to have these products if they are part of a cooked dish, such as a casserole, however.
- Raw (unpasteurized) milk or foods that contain unpasteurized milk.

Toxoplasmosis

Toxoplasmosis is caused by a parasite known as *Toxoplasma gondii* (or *T. gondii*). If you become pregnant while you have toxoplasmosis (which means that *T. gondii* is roaming your bloodstream), the parasite can pass through the placenta and harm your unborn child. In babies, toxoplasmosis is capable of causing hearing loss, mental retardation, and blindness. Some children who are born to mothers with toxoplasmosis can develop brain or eye problems years after birth. If a pregnant woman contracts toxoplasmosis, there's a 50 percent chance she'll pass it on to her child.

Raw or undercooked meat is the predominant source of *T. gondii.* Other sources are unwashed fruits and vegetables, contaminated water, dust, soil, dirty kitty-litter boxes, and outdoor areas where cat feces are found. If you have a cat that goes outdoors and you're thinking about becoming pregnant or are pregnant, you may be at risk for toxoplasmosis. That's because *T. gondii* infects just about all cats that spend any time out of the house. Since *T. gondii* doesn't make your cat sick, you probably won't know if your pet harbors the parasite.

You can become exposed to *T. gondii* by an accidental ingestion of contaminated cat feces. This might sound improbable, but it can inadvertently occur if you touch your unwashed hands to your mouth after you've been gardening, cleaning a litter box, or touching anything that comes in contact with cat feces. Over time, typically about a week, the parasite can enter your bloodstream.

Like listeriosis, toxoplasmosis can be difficult to detect; only about 10 percent of women who are infected with the parasite have noticeable symptoms. These can include swollen glands, fever, headache, muscle pain, or a stiff neck. Get tested for toxoplasmosis before conceiving, or if you experience any of the above symptoms. If you are infected, you can take medication to clear your body of *T. gondii*. However, you'll have to wait for six months after the infection clears up to become pregnant.

You can greatly reduce your risk for toxoplasmosis by avoiding raw or undercooked meat and unwashed fruits and vegetables. If you have a cat, you should change the litter box daily (the parasite does not become infectious for one to five days after it has been shed in the feces) or have someone else change it. Wear gloves when you're cleaning the litter box and when you're gardening or handling sand from a sandbox; cover sandboxes whenever possible to keep cats out. Don't get a new cat when you're pregnant.

E. Coli Infections

E. coli infections are typically caused by *Escherichia coli* O157:H7, the most powerful of hundreds of strains of the bacterium *Escherichia coli*. *Escherichia coli* O157:H7 is a leading suspect when food-borne illness occurs. Undercooked or raw beef tainted with the bacteria is often the cause of E. coli infections. You can become infected with E. coli from consuming contaminated bean sprouts, fresh leafy greens like lettuce and spinach, and unpasteurized (raw) milk and juices.

If you get an E. coli infection, you will experience abdominal cramps and bloody diarrhea two to eight days after ingesting the tainted food. An E. coli infection is very serious in young children if it causes hemolytic uremic syndrome, in which the body's red blood cells are destroyed and the kidneys can fail. Most healthy people, however, recover from E. coli infections within ten days.

Salmonella Poisoning

Salmonella poisoning is caused by the genus *Salmonella*, a group of bacteria. The symptoms of salmonella poisoning are diarrhea, fever, and abdominal cramps that begin twelve to seventy-two hours after exposure. Most of the time, salmonella poisoning lasts about seven days, and there are no permanent side effects.

Some people—especially those with weakened immune systems, pregnant women, and small children—are prone to a severe form of salmonellosis and may need to be hospitalized and given antibiotics to cure a salmonella infection. A small percentage of people infected with *Salmonella* develop Reiter's syndrome, a condition characterized by joint pain, eye irritation, and painful urination. Reiter's syndrome can last for months or years, resulting in chronic arthritis.

Foods contaminated by *Salmonella* usually look and smell normal. Animal foods, such as beef, poultry, raw milk, or raw eggs, are more likely to contain *Salmonella,* but all foods, including vegetables, are prone to contamination. Proper cooking typically kills the bacteria.

Simple Steps to Safer Food

Although troubling germs lurk in the food we eat, most food, when handled properly, is perfectly safe. Err on the side of caution with these five basic steps to food safety.

Shop Wisely

Make sure that all of the food you buy is in good condition. Meat, poultry, and dairy foods should be as fresh as possible; check the expiration or sell-by date to be sure. Pick up the cold and frozen foods on your list, such as meat and dairy products, from the grocery store shelves last, just before you head for the checkout. Go directly home and put the refrigerated and frozen foods away immediately, to preserve freshness. Use ready-to-eat, highly perishable foods, such as dairy products, meat, seafood, and produce, as soon as possible after you buy them.

Keep Hands and Utensils Clean

Before you handle food, always wash your hands thoroughly (for at least twenty seconds) with warm soapy water. Wash them again during food preparation if you have wiped your nose, coughed, or sneezed into your hand, used the bathroom, changed a diaper, handled dirty laundry, touched a pet, taken out the garbage, or performed any other activity that could transfer germs to your hands. Other people's germs can make you sick, so encourage proper hand washing by your family and guests by making soap and clean towels or paper towels available at every sink in your home. When you can't use soap, rely on alcohol-based wipes or gel formulas, which are effective for sanitizing the hands.

Clean your cutting boards, dishes, utensils, and countertops thoroughly with dishwashing soap or a cleaning agent that is safe to use on surfaces that come in contact with food. Replace worn cutting boards (including plastic, nonporous acrylic, and wooden boards), because bacteria can grow in the hard-to-clean grooves and cracks.

Always rinse raw fruits and vegetables under cold running water before using them. For thick or rough-skinned vegetables and fruits (such as potatoes, carrots, and cantaloupe), use a small vegetable brush to remove the surface dirt. Cut away the damaged or bruised areas on produce, because germs thrive in these moist places.

Good Germs, Bad Germs

An obsession with cleanliness has led to a boom in antimicrobial soaps and hand washes in order to remove the germs from our lives. The irony is that in our quest to rid germs, we could be doing more harm than good by helping the remaining bacteria to build up a resistance to antibiotics. This may come as a surprise, but some bacteria are actually good for you. However, antimicrobial soaps and other cleansing agents cannot discriminate between good and bad bacteria, so they kill them all. Do your immune system a favor: stick with regular soap and water. Here's another helpful hint to keep bad bacteria at bay. Sanitize your kitchen countertops with this homemade cleanser: mix one teaspoon of liquid chlorine bleach in a quart of clean water. Wipe countertops and cutting boards with the bleach solution and leave it for about ten minutes, before rinsing, for maximum effect.

Keep Certain Foods Separate

Segregate raw animal foods, such as meat, seafood, and eggs, from ready-to-eat foods, like salad greens and chopped fruit. Use a separate plate for cooked food. For example, when you're grilling meats or seafood, do not use the same platter, plate, or bowl for the cooked meat or fish that you used for marinating the raw meat or fish.

Cook Food Properly

Cooking destroys harmful germs, but only when the food has been heated to the proper temperature. Have a reliable meat thermometer on hand, and cook (and reheat) foods properly, using these handy guidelines.

Cook fish until it reaches an internal temperature of 145°F (63°C). If you don't have a food thermometer or it's not appropriate to use one, cook the fish until it flakes with a fork. Allow shrimp, lobster, and scallops to reach the appropriate color: shrimp should be pink and the flesh opaque (milky white); properly cooked lobster meat and scallops will be opaque, too, as well as firm to the touch. Cook clams, mussels, and oysters just until their shells open. Discard shellfish with closed shells.

Here's a list of cooking temperatures for meats and eggs for easy reference:

Type of Meat	Cook to at Least
Whole poultry (chicken or turkey; take temperature in thigh)	180°F (82°C)
Chicken or turkey breast	170°F (77°C)
Ground chicken or turkey	165°F (74°C)
Ground beef, veal, lamb, and pork	160°F (71°C)
Pork roasts and chops	145°F (63°C)

Cook eggs until the yolks and whites are firm. Let egg dishes reach 160°F (71°C). Do not eat raw or partially cooked eggs in any form.

Reheat all leftovers to 165°F (74°C). Bring leftover soups, sauces, and gravy to a boil. If you won't be arriving home within two hours of being served at a restaurant, don't take leftovers or any other food with you. When you order takeout, eat the food immediately or refrigerate it right away.

When Raw Is Risky

You've been eating sushi for years without a problem. Maybe you always order your favorite sandwich with raw sprouts. Perhaps you adore raw oysters or steak tartare. When a pregnancy is in your future or is happening now, however, you might want to think twice the next time you decide what to eat.

Raw or undercooked fish, including sushi and sashimi, are more likely than properly cooked fish to contain parasites and bacteria. Raw shellfish (oysters, clams, mussels) is one of the worst offenders for potentially making you sick, so avoid it. The same is true for raw or undercooked meat and eggs.

Sprouts are good for you, but they should be cooked. Alfalfa, clover, radish, and other sprouts are highly susceptible to bacterial contamination that cannot be washed off, for the most part. In addition, stay away from unpasteurized juice and milk and from dishes that are made with raw eggs, such as Caesar salad and homemade eggnog.

Refrigerate Perishables

Most bacteria thrive from 40°F (4°C) to 140°F (60°C). Discourage growth by keeping your refrigerator at 40°F (4°C) or below and the freezer at 0°F (−18°C). Use a refrigerator thermometer, and check the temperature periodically. Don't pack the refrigerator too full with food. Cold air must circulate to keep food safe.

Refrigerate or freeze perishables, prepared food, and leftovers within two hours of eating them or preparing them. It's fine to place warm or hot food in the refrigerator; doing so won't harm the food or your refrigerator. Be sure to divide large amounts of leftovers into shallow containers for quicker cooling in the refrigerator. Discard food that's been left out at room temperature (about 70°F or 21°C) for longer than two hours. When the air temperature registers 90°F or above (32°C), pitch the food after one hour.

At outdoor events, use a cooler to keep cold foods cold. Fill the cooler with food and ice or cold packs. A full cooler maintains its cold temperature longer than one that's only partly filled.

Marinades, Microwaves, and Defrosting

Marinating is a great way to tenderize meat or seafood while also adding flavor, but you must be careful with marinades. Never reuse a marinade on cooked foods unless you boil it first. Always marinate foods in the refrigerator—not at room temperature.

Microwave ovens tend to heat foods unevenly, leaving some cold spots where bacteria can thrive. Fat, fluid, and sugar heat more quickly, so be careful not to burn yourself. Microwaving vegetables makes preparation a snap. When you add some liquid to the microwavable dish and cover, you create steam that kills bacteria. Ensure even heating by turning the dish several times and stirring soups and stews periodically.

If you defrost food in the microwave, cook the food right away to prevent bacterial growth. Bear in mind that some areas of the food may become warm and begin to cook during defrosting, allowing germs to thrive. Cooking right away helps to prevent bacterial growth.

If you don't use the microwave to defrost food, you have two other safe choices. Defrost in the refrigerator or in cold water, changing the water every thirty minutes to keep it cold. Don't defrost foods on the counter or anywhere else at room temperature. Any bacteria present in the food will quickly begin to reproduce.

Seafood Safety

You're a seafood lover. You adore fried clams and baked scallops, and you never pass up a chance to order a swordfish steak when dining out. Perhaps you would eat a tuna fish sandwich every day, given the opportunity.

Seafood is an important part of a balanced eating plan. Fish and shellfish pack high-quality protein, vitamins, and minerals. Though relatively low in total fat, fish and shellfish provide omega-3 fats, which play a pivotal role in your future child's vision and brain development.

However, certain fish harbor high levels of methylmercury, which accumulates in your body and can harm your child once you conceive. Other potential fish contaminants include dioxins and polychlorinated biphenyls (PCBs), chemicals once used by industry in the United States.

Mercury

Methylmercury is the most dangerous type of mercury. It's formed when mercury that is emitted into the air from coal-burning power plants and other industrial activity gets into bodies of water. Bacteria that live in oceans, lakes, and other water convert mercury to methylmercury. Fish then absorb the methylmercury from their food supply in these contaminated waters.

Certain large, ocean fish harbor the most methylmercury. The Food and Drug Administration (FDA) warns women in their childbearing years to avoid swordfish, tilefish, king mackerel, and shark because of their excessive methylmercury content.

Even if you're not pregnant, you should still be concerned about methylmercury. Methylmercury accumulates in your bodily tissues and is capable of passing from your blood into that of your unborn child, wreaking havoc on a baby's developing nervous system.

Other chemicals in fish are also a concern. Game fish—any fish caught for sport, such as trout or bass—may also be contaminated with industrial pollutants, including PCBs. Some studies suggest that a developing baby's exposure to PCBs contributes to a lower birth weight, learning problems, and decreased IQ. If you eat fish caught for sport, check the safety of the rivers, lakes, and streams where the fish has been caught. Contact your local or state health department to find out if the waters are safe.

Making Wise Choices

Despite the warnings about fish, there's no need to completely avoid it when you're trying to conceive or during pregnancy and nursing. In spite of the concerns about mercury, there is evidence to suggest that it might not be as problematic as people think. Selenium, a mineral that is plentiful in cold-water seafood such as salmon, may help to protect your body from methylmercury contamination.

The Avon Longitudinal Study on Parents and Children, a recent eight-year study of about twelve thousand women and their children, underscores the importance of seafood in the diets of pregnant women. The children of pregnant women who consumed more than twelve ounces a week of any type of fish benefited the most. These children scored higher on measures of academic prowess at age eight and had fewer behavioral and social difficulties earlier in life than children born to mothers who ate less than twelve ounces of fish a week during pregnancy.

The researchers did not measure the levels of mercury and other contaminants in the seafood the pregnant women ate, but they concluded that the fish consumed by the women in the study, which was done in Britain, was unlikely to have been lower in methylmercury than what the general U.S. population would eat if it was consuming the same amounts of seafood. Britain does have lower PCB contamination levels than other developed countries, however, including the United States.

To reap the benefits of seafood, choose a variety of fish that is considered safe to eat. It's perfectly fine to eat up to twelve ounces (two average meals) a week of fish and shellfish that are lower in mercury, including the following:

- Shrimp
- Canned light tuna (limit albacore, or white, tuna to 6 ounces weekly, however)
- Salmon (farmed or wild)
- Sardines
- Pollock
- Catfish
- Tilapia

For a longer list of the safest fish to eat during your childbearing years, visit the Environmental Working Group's Web site at www.ewg .org/safefishlist.

Lead

The Environmental Protection Agency banned the use of lead in gasoline, paint, and many other products in the 1970s. Nevertheless, even though environmental lead levels are on the decline, this toxic metal lingers.

Lead in your body can wreak havoc on the development of your child's brain and central nervous system. Young children and unborn babies run the greatest risk of damage when exposed to lead. During pregnancy, exposure to excessive lead can cause low birth weight, preterm delivery, developmental delays in infants, and miscarriage. Even low levels of lead exposure can cause learning and behavioral problems in children.

You may come into contact with lead if you or anyone in your household works in an auto repair shop, a battery manufacturing plant, or certain types of construction. To minimize your lead exposure, have the people you live with who work at those jobs change their clothes before coming into the house. Wash their clothes separately from yours.

Older houses may contain lead-based paint. Pregnant women and small children must not live or stay in the house while lead paint is being removed or being sanded or scraped. Drinking water can pose another lead risk. Lead from lead pipes can leach into drinking water, and so can the lead solder on copper pipes and brass faucets. Many home water filters do not remove lead from the water. Testing is the only way to confirm if lead is present in your home's drinking water.

Lead is bad news, but a balanced diet can help to prevent lead accumulation in bone tissue. Be sure to get enough calcium, zinc, and iron on a low-fat eating plan to guard against lead contamination. Blood lead levels should measure 10 micrograms per deciliter (mcg/dl) or less prior to pregnancy and breast-feeding in order to reduce a child's contact with lead. If you're at all concerned about the level of lead in your body, request a blood test from your health-care provider.

What's in Your Water?

Most water systems test for lead as a regular part of water monitoring. These tests give a systemwide picture and do not reflect the conditions at a specific drinking water outlet, however. For more information on testing your water, call the Environmental Protection Agency's Safe Drinking Water Hotline at 1-800-426-4791. The National Lead Information Center, at www.epa.gov/lead, is helpful, too.

Endocrine Disruptors

Your endocrine system is a complicated network of hormones and glands, such as the thyroid, the pituitary gland, and the ovaries. The endocrine system regulates many bodily functions, including reproduction.

Endocrine disruptors are chemicals that include certain types of dioxins, a class of compounds that are by-products of industrial processes that involve chlorine, such as the bleaching of everyday items like coffee filters, and PCBs. PCBs are a category of chemicals that were used to insulate or cool electrical transformers, that were part of hydraulic fluid, and that functioned as lubricants for machinery. PCBs were banned from use by the U.S. government in the 1970s, but, like lead, they remain in the environment.

Endocrine disruptors are compounds that fool the body into responding at the wrong time or that block the effects of a natural hormone, such as estrogen or testosterone. In fact, endocrine disruptors are capable of mimicking estrogen and affecting testosterone levels at crucial times of development during pregnancy.

You can cut down on your exposure to endocrine disruptors in food by choosing lean meats and low-fat or fat-free dairy products. That's because harmful chemicals congregate most often in fat tissue. Avoid eating contaminated fish. Consult your local or state health department about which bodies of water are considered unsafe for fishing. Peel the skin off fruits and vegetables whenever possible, because chemicals build up in their skins as they grow.

Should You Go Organic?

Organic milk, meat, and produce are growing in popularity. You know that organic food, typically thought of as chemical-free by many consumers, is probably better for you, yet it's pricey. Even though cost-conscious stores such as Wal-Mart sell organic fare, it can take a bite out of your food budget. Whether you should spend the extra money for organic foods depends on a number of factors.

What's in a Label?

A product label with the U.S. Department of Agriculture's (USDA) organic seal will say either "100% organic" or just "organic," which means that the product contains 95 percent to 100 percent organic ingredients. Foods that contain a minimum of 70 percent but less than 95 percent organic ingredients will read "made with organic ingredients" but cannot display the USDA seal. "Natural" is not the same as organic. A "natural" claim has no legal definition.

Organic produce is grown without synthetic pesticides or synthetic fertilizers and without sewage sludge (yes, you read that right). Organic fruits and vegetables have not been genetically engineered or radiated to kill bacteria and parasites. Organic beef and poultry are from animals that were raised on 100 percent organic feed and were never given growth hormones, antibiotics, or any other drugs. Organic beef and poultry cannot come from cloned animals and may not be radiated. Eggs labeled organic are from hens that are fed 100 percent organic feed and have never been given antibiotics or growth hormones.

Remember, though, that just because a product is organic, it's not necessarily good for you. Many processed organic foods, such as cookies and chips, are high in calories and fat as well as sodium and sugar.

Produce

Organic produce is raised without synthetic fertilizers or synthetic pesticides. In comparison, hundreds of man-made pesticides—chemicals that defend crops from pests that would ruin them—are used on conventional produce in the United States.

It's hard to say how much harm is caused by the synthetic pesticides and other contaminants in conventional produce, because there is little data available on the safety of most pesticides. Even harder to figure out is the danger of long-term exposure to low levels of a combination of chemicals used in food, which is more typical of the exposure you get from eating fruits and vegetables. It's also next to impossible to sort out the damage done by food pesticide residues and the tiny amounts of hundreds of other chemicals you're exposed to every day in the general environment.

Nevertheless, when you are of childbearing age, pregnant, or nursing, it's a good idea to avoid as many synthetic pesticides as possible. Pesticides and other chemicals in food and the environment may be detrimental, especially during vulnerable periods of life, including fetal development and early childhood, when exposure can have long-lasting effects.

Studies of large groups of people have found lower rates of heart disease and certain cancers in those who were consuming the most fruits and vegetables. The evidence that produce is a powerful weapon against certain chronic conditions is so convincing that experts say it's more beneficial to your health to eat conventional fruits and vegetables than to go without adequate amounts of produce.

It still makes sense to limit chemical exposure as much as possible, however. Buying organic produce can minimize, but not completely eliminate, the risk of pesticide residues; this might come as a surprise to people who are currently spending the extra money for organic foods. Small amounts of pesticide residues are unavoidable even on many organic fruits and vegetables, because wind and water spread pesticides that have been used on other crops. Furthermore, some pesticides persist in the soil for years and are absorbed by plants long after the land has been certified organic. Nevertheless, organic produce harbors much lower levels of pesticides. See the section "When to Be Picky" below for information on how to reduce pesticide consumption.

Organically produced meat, milk, eggs, fruit, vegetables, and grains do not provide automatic protection from E. coli infections, salmonella poisoning, or other food-borne hazards. Organic foods, including unpasteurized juice and milk, have just as much (or more, if they are unpasteurized) chance as nonorganic foods of harboring the harmful germs that cause these conditions, so handle organic fare with care.

Although there is some evidence that foods grown and produced without the use of synthetic fertilizers and pesticides are higher in nutrients, there is no appreciable difference.

Reduce the Risk

Washing and rinsing fresh produce may lower the level of some pesticides, but it won't completely eliminate them. Peeling also reduces the pesticide level, but valuable nutrients often go down the drain with the peel. To reduce your risk, eat a variety of foods; wash produce thoroughly; pick organic foods, if possible; and choose conventional fruits and vegetables with the lowest levels of chemical contaminants.

When to Be Picky

Organic food costs more, so you may not be able to go completely organic. Don't worry; you probably don't need to do so. There are some conventional foods that you might want to choose to avoid, however.

The Environmental Working Group (EWG), a nonprofit consumer protection agency, based the determination of the twelve cleanest fruits and vegetables and the dirtiest dozen (the most contaminated) on nearly forty-three thousand tests for pesticides on produce collected by the USDA and the FDA between 2000 and 2005. However, the assessment did not account for the toxicity of each of the pesticides, which is difficult to determine. The two following lists are from the EWG's *Shopper's Guide to Pesticides in Produce* (visit www.ewg.org for more information).

There's no need to go organic for these twelve fruits and vegetables, which came out consistently low in pesticide residues, according to the EWG's analysis.

Onions	Avocado
Cabbage	Pineapples
Broccoli	Mangoes
Asparagus	Papaya
Sweet peas (frozen)	Kiwi
Sweet corn (frozen)	Bananas

The EWG estimates that you can cut your pesticide exposure by as much as 90 percent by avoiding what it considers to be the most contaminated produce, which includes the following twelve foods:

Peaches	Grapes (imported)
Nectarines	Bell peppers
Pears	Celery
Apples	Spinach
Strawberries	Lettuce
Cherries	Potatoes

Milk

Organic milk is identified by the official USDA certified organic seal. It comes from cows that have been fed an organic diet for at least the past year or during their entire lives, and they have also not been given growth hormones or antibiotics. "Hormone-free milk" does not mean organic. There is no such thing as truly hormone-free milk. That's because milk, even the organic variety, contains, at the very least, low levels of bovine somatotropin (BST), also called bovine growth hormone (BGH), which is produced naturally by cows. Recombinant BST (rBST) is a bioengineered version of natural BST that is given to cows to boost milk production. Milk from cows given rBST is safe, according to the FDA. The use of rBST is not an issue with certified organic milk, because the criteria state that organic milk cannot come from cows treated with rBST. However, if the milk is not organic, then the cow it came from could have been given antibiotics as well as rBST.

Pesticide residues are uncommon in milk.

Meat and Seafood

Certified organic livestock isn't given antibiotics unless an animal is sick. The animals eat 100 percent certified organic feed or grass that's been grown without toxic pesticides or fertilizers. Don't count on free-range animals, however; free-range provides no guarantee that the meat or poultry from those animals is antibiotic-free. Pesticide residues are uncommon in beef, poultry, and eggs. If pesticides are present, they reside in the animal's fat. Reduce the risk of exposure by choosing lower-fat cuts of meat.

Don't bother with so-called organic seafood—there are no government standards for it.

Grains

When you're buying refined grains, such as white bread, certain crackers, and white rice, save your money. Any pesticides are largely stripped away during the processing, when the bran part of the grain is removed. It's best to purchase organic whole grains, however. That's because the grain is intact, and whole grains tend to be richer in fiber, vitamins, minerals, and phytonutrients.

Food Additives

When you're unfamiliar with the lingo, studying the ingredients on food labels is like trying to decipher a foreign language, with words like *niacinamide, pyridoxine hydrochloride, ferrous gluconate,* and *ascorbic acid* staring back at you. Even though the names are difficult to decode, most food additives are considered safe, including the ones mentioned above, which are the scientific monikers for common vitamins and minerals.

There are several reasons for adding anything to food. Some additives, like vitamin C, foster freshness; others, like sugar and salt, enhance taste and appearance; still others boost nutrition that was lost in processing. For example, B vitamins that were stripped away during the making of refined grains, like white bread, are added back in, resulting in an *enriched* product. *Fortified* foods, on the other hand, contain nutrients that were not present naturally. Most milk is fortified with vitamins A and D, for instance. Iron is often added to breads, cereal, and other grains to enhance their nutritional profile.

Most additives are safe, but some have pitfalls. The sulfites that are used on fresh produce, on dried fruit, and in commercial bread products may trigger allergies in some people with asthma. Sodium nitrate and sodium nitrite, which provide hot dogs and other cured meats with their pink hue and protect them from germ growth, are potential carcinogens. Avoid the preservatives BHA and BHT; they too are suspected cancer-starters.

If you want to limit food additives, eat a diet that is rich in fresh and lightly processed foods. Following that advice will also curb your consumption of salt and sugar, which are common food additives. Foods labeled "preservative-free" contain fewer food additives.

Better Safe Than Sorry

Reading about the germs and other contaminants in food and water can be very scary. It's necessary to alert women of childbearing age to the dangers from food in order to protect them and their future children. Try not to be alarmed, however. Overall, our food supply is very safe. Armed with just a few basics, it's possible for you to help everyone in your family avoid becoming ill from food and water.

7

Infertility, Other Common Concerns, and Special Situations

Some couples find it difficult to conceive, and many women face more than their fair share of discomfort during pregnancy. Some have complications that put their pregnancy at risk, whereas others have relatively little to contend with for nine months. Here are some of the most common issues that face pregnant women and their partners as well as some ideas on how to manage or minimize them with diet and lifestyle.

The Age Factor

You can't change how old you are. For most women having babies, however, age matters little to their health or to their baby's. For other pregnant women, their age makes healthy diet and lifestyle habits even more important.

Young and Pregnant

Teen mothers become pregnant before their bodies have had a chance to fully mature. The irony is that even though they are able to conceive a child, teens are just barely on the verge of adulthood themselves. Pregnant teens may not meet their elevated nutrient needs, particularly for iron and calcium. That's because many adolescents make poor food choices, preferring soft drinks to milk; french fries to baked potatoes; and fast food instead of more nutritious, homemade fare. Young people also tend to skip meals more often than older people do. As a result, a teen mother-to-be and her growing baby may end up competing for nutrients, shortchanging both in terms of health and development.

More Calcium, Better Bones

Adolescence is when teens accumulate much of the bone mass they will have for life. According to the Institute of Medicine, pregnant teens don't need additional calcium. A study from the Center for Human Nutrition at the Johns Hopkins Bloomberg School of Public Health suggests otherwise, however. Extra calcium may be the ticket for building bone mass during this vulnerable time of life. Researchers examined the effect of teen pregnancy on bone health in thirteen- to eighteen-year-old mothers and found that one-third of the young mothers had a bone mass that qualified as osteoporosis, or osteopenia (the prelude to osteoporosis), shortly after pregnancy. Girls who consumed more calcium during pregnancy showed less bone loss when tested after delivering than girls with poor or average calcium intakes did.

Teens tend to enter pregnancy at an unhealthy weight more often than their older counterparts, and they are less likely to gain the recommended number of pounds. Adolescent mothers are more prone to deliver pre-term babies (before thirty-seven weeks), experience anemia, and have elevated blood pressure.

Because teens in general often fail to satisfy the quotas for important nutrients such as protein, iron, and calcium, it's difficult to imagine that they would be able to meet the much higher levels that pregnancy demands. However, it is possible to have a healthy baby and nourish a teen body at the same time. If you're a teenage mother-to-be, take your diet and lifestyle seriously. Here are some healthy strategies for doing just that:

- Seek regular prenatal care as soon as possible after you find out you're pregnant.
- Take a prescription prenatal vitamin and mineral pill every day. You may need extra supplements, such as calcium, iron, and doco-sahexaenoic acid (DHA). Discuss your nutrient needs with your health-care provider or with a registered dietitian (RD).
- Read chapter 3 to help you plan the healthiest diet possible. If you need help, consult an RD to devise an eating plan that's tailored to meet your needs. Get a free referral to a dietitian in your area by going to www.eatright.org, the Web site of the American Dietetic Association. Or check out the government's Special Supplement Program for Women, Infants and Children, better known as WIC, for assistance. This program serves low-income pregnant and breast-feeding women and their children up to age five, and provides nutritious foods, nutrition education, and referrals to health services and other organizations, free of charge. Visit www. fns.usda.gov for the location of an office in your area.
- Eat on a regular basis throughout the day, having at least three balanced meals. Try to work in foods from at least two of the five food groups in each snack and foods from at least three food groups at each meal.
- Avoid too much caffeine and all alcohol. See chapter 2 for more information on how much caffeine is safe during pregnancy and nursing.
- Stop smoking, and do not use illegal (recreational) drugs.
- Speak with your doctor or pharmacist about any medications and herbal supplements you take, even if just occasionally. They may be harmful to your unborn child.

The Older Mother

You might have had your last child more than five years ago and now find yourself pregnant again at thirty-five, forty, or forty-two. Maybe you're trying for your first baby later in life. You're not alone. Preliminary data from the Centers for Disease Control and Prevention for 2006 suggest that the birth rate of mothers ages thirty-five to thirty-nine is the highest it's been since 1964. Women aged forty to forty-four are giving birth at a rate unsurpassed since 1968.

Age has its advantages and its disadvantages. If you already have a family, you know what to expect from pregnancy and childbirth. Each pregnancy is unique, but this pregnancy may be harder on your body. Although many older women experience few complications and deliver healthy babies, the passage of time means that you're more likely to be managing pregnancy in addition to a health condition, such as type 2 diabetes, high blood pressure, or being overweight. That makes paying attention to your special dietary and lifestyle needs more important than ever.

You may have more trouble conceiving after age thirty-five, but when you do conceive, you're more likely to have twins, so be prepared to get more than you might have expected. Having more than one child after the age of thirty-five presents even more of a health challenge because of the added strain on your body.

If this is your first pregnancy and you're older than thirty-five, it's particularly important for you to seek preconception care to manage any health problems you might have before conception. Other than that, the lifestyle advice for healthy older mothers is pretty much the same as for a mother in her twenties or early thirties.

Multiple Births

Though still relatively low, the rate of multiple births has risen steadily in the last two decades. Most women who have multiple births deliver twins. About one-third of the increase in the incidence of multiple births in the last few decades is due to the fact that more women over the age of thirty are having children. Older women are more likely to conceive multiple babies. The remainder of the increase in multiple births is due to assisted reproductive techniques such as in vitro fertilization. Nearly half of assisted pregnancies result in twins; 7 percent yield triplets or in rare cases, quadruplets, quintuplets, sextuplets, or septuplets.

In addition to the telltale heartbeats heard on an ultrasound device, there are some other signs that you're having a multiple birth, including rapid weight gain during the first trimester, a larger-than-expected uterus, and severe morning sickness.

Multiple pregnancies tend to be shorter than singleton pregnancies, and they also tend to be more complicated. When you're expecting two or more babies, there's more of a chance that you'll develop preeclampsia (see page 185) and gestational diabetes (see page 182). Most twins do not make it to forty weeks of gestation, and more than 90 percent of triplets don't, either. On average, twins are born at thirty-five weeks, triplets at thirty-three weeks, and an uncomplicated singleton at 39 weeks. Because multiple pregnancies don't typically go full-term, they can result in low-birth-weight babies. Low-birth-weight babies tend to have more medical problems immediately after birth and throughout life.

If you are having multiple babies, expect to see your health-care provider more often than if you were pregnant with only one child. To properly monitor the progress of your pregnancy, you may need an appointment twice a month in your second trimester and weekly in the third trimester.

Weight gain will also be different. If you began pregnancy with a BMI of between 19.8 and 26 (see chapter 1), you'll be encouraged to gain thirty-five to forty-five pounds for twins, or about one pound per week in the first twenty weeks of pregnancy and just over a pound a week for the duration of the pregnancy. To gain that many pounds, you'll probably need to eat about 500 extra calories a day beyond your prepregnancy energy needs, starting as soon as you get a positive pregnancy test. Women who are pregnant with triplets may need to eat even more than 500 additional calories every day to gain enough weight. Speak to your health-care provider about how many pounds you should gain.

Healthy food choices are particularly important when you're having more than one child. For example, a twin pregnancy requires fifty grams more protein each day; that's twenty-five more than what a woman who is having one child needs. See chapter 2 for more about satisfying your daily protein quota.

Having multiple babies may produce serious morning sickness that prevents you from taking your prescription prenatal vitamin pill every day. Try everything you can to work in those extra nutrients, including talking with your health-care provider about the most palatable forms of dietary supplements, including chewable prenatal vitamins. Adequate iron is especially critical in multiple pregnancies. Iron-deficiency anemia, which can increase the risk of preterm delivery, is more common in women who are having multiple babies.

Constipation

Constipation is generally defined as moving your bowels three or fewer times a week. When you have constipation, your stools are usually hard, dry, and small in size. Some people who are constipated find it painful to have a bowel movement and often experience straining, bloating, and the sensation of full bowels.

Constipation can set in as early as the first trimester. The pregnancy hormone progesterone may be to blame, because it slows the movement of food through your digestive tract. Taking large doses of iron, such as in prenatal pills and other dietary supplements, can cause constipation, too. As your pregnancy progresses, your expanding uterus puts pressure on your intestines, which contributes to constipation.

Constipation is common following childbirth and surgery. Delivery is hard on the muscles that are used to pass a stool. Your bowels may also be sluggish because of the drugs and anesthetics you received during delivery. You may feel particularly gassy if you're recovering from a cesarean section.

The sooner your intestinal tract is in top working order, the better. Here's how to curb constipation:

- **Focus on fiber.** Fiber-rich foods, such as fruits, vegetables, legumes, and whole grains, bulk up stools, making them easy to pass. Aim for at least 28 grams of fiber a day. See chapter 2 for more on fiber sources and fiber needs. Start increasing your fiber intake slowly to avoid gas and bloating.

> WORDS OF
> *Motherly Wisdom*
>
> "I found that including a high-fiber cereal every day, avoiding too much cheese (it can be binding), and munching on dried fruit and nuts works to relieve constipation."
> —Dina

- **Drink up.** Liquids add fluid to the colon, which promotes bulkier and softer stools. Pregnant women need at least ten eight-ounce glasses of fluid daily, and nursing women need thirteen; if you're not nursing, aim for nine glasses.
- **Work it out.** Physical activity increases the flow of blood, which can help prevent constipation.

Hemorrhoids

Constipation is bad enough, but if you then strained to move your bowels, you may have acquired hemorrhoids, which are swollen veins in the rectal area that can become itchy or painful and might bleed. To make matters worse, pregnancy hormones enable the walls of your veins to relax and swell more easily. Pressure on your intestinal tract from a growing baby can bring on hemorrhoids, too; so can sitting or standing for long periods. In addition, pushing during labor can cause hemorrhoids.

If you had hemorrhoids before, you're more prone to get them during pregnancy. To add insult to injury, developing hemorrhoids during one delivery increases the risk of a flare-up during future pregnancies. Hemorrhoids are manageable, however. Following the advice for avoiding constipation is a good place to start—before, during, and after pregnancy. When you're expecting, stick to the weight-gain guidelines that are right for you; extra weight exacerbates hemorrhoids.

Ask your doctor or other health-care professional how to manage the discomfort of hemorrhoids. Always check with your provider before using any medication to ease the pain and swelling that hemorrhoids provoke.

Heartburn

In spite of the name, heartburn has nothing to do with your heart. *Acid indigestion* is a better moniker for this sour, burning sensation in the upper abdomen, the chest, or the throat.

Stomach acid is at the root of heartburn. When gastric juices stay where they belong—in the stomach—they pose no problem. Heartburn happens when stomach acid splashes into the esophagus, the tube that carries food from your mouth to your stomach. This backwash occurs because of too-frequent relaxation of the lower esophageal sphincter, a muscular valve that separates the esophagus and the stomach. When the sphincter relaxes, it allows the stomach acid to move upward into the esophagus, causing symptoms of heartburn and, in severe cases, damage to the esophageal lining.

Changing hormone levels during pregnancy can generate heartburn, because they relax the muscles of the digestive tract and also influence how you tolerate food. Pregnant women are susceptible to heartburn at any time, but it's common in the third trimester, when the baby is big enough to crowd your stomach and push stomach contents into the esophagus. About half of all pregnant women have heartburn in the latter part of pregnancy, according to the American College of Gastroenterology.

When Heartburn Hangs On

Frequent bouts of heartburn after delivery has come and gone may be a sign of something more serious than discomfort. If you have heartburn two or more times a week, you could have gastroesophageal reflux disease (GERD). Treating GERD protects your esophageal lining from damage that could eventually give rise to cancer. Managing GERD may be as simple as taking over-the-counter medications or prescription drugs. Sometimes, however, GERD requires surgery. Let your doctor know if you are nursing a child so that the appropriate medication can be prescribed, if necessary.

Try these techniques to put out the fire in your belly:

- Eat smaller meals throughout the day instead of larger ones, especially at dinner. When you make a meal, eat half and save the rest for a few hours later.
- Chew your food completely for better digestion. Don't rush your meals.
- Avoid known stomach irritants, including spicy tomato foods, fried foods and other fatty fare, chocolate, carbonated beverages, caffeine, and anything else that bothers you.
- Drink fluids between meals, not with them. Too many fluids with food can crowd your stomach and encourage reflux.

- Sit up after eating. Prop your head up in bed to prevent stomach acids from reaching chest level at night. Wait at least an hour after eating to go to bed.
- Chew gum. Chewing stimulates the swallowing of saliva, which buffers acid in the esophagus.

If these measures fail, consult your doctor about medications such as Tums or Maalox; chewable forms adhere best to esophageal tissue, where they provide relief. However, do not take any medication to mitigate heartburn without checking first with your health-care provider.

When You Can't Get Pregnant: The Connections among Diet, Lifestyle, and Infertility

If you and your partner have been trying to conceive for at least a year (or six months if you're older than thirty-five), but it's not working, you may be experiencing infertility.

There are many reasons for the infertility that affects about seven million couples in the United States. About one-third of infertility cases are traceable to the woman, another one-third to the man, and another one-third to a combination of problems in both partners. Some cases of infertility are inexplicable.

Ovulation disorders, including polycystic ovary syndrome (see the next section) are the most common culprits in curbing female fertility. Other causes are pelvic inflammatory disease and endometriosis.

Focus on Fertility

A woman's ability to become pregnant is influenced by a number of lifestyle and environmental factors, including the following:

- Her age, and her partner's
- Stress
- Poor diet
- Being overweight or underweight
- Smoking cigarettes and using recreational drugs or alcohol
- Medication
- Environmental toxins, such as perchloroethylene (dry cleaning fluid) and lead, found in drinking water and other places

---

Polycystic Ovary Syndrome

Polycystic ovary syndrome (PCOS) affects about 10 percent of women in their childbearing years. It's the number one reason for infertility in women. PCOS causes menstrual irregularities and can wreak havoc with your hormones, heart, blood vessels, and appearance. No one is exactly sure what causes PCOS, but experts suspect that insulin resistance is the primary factor. Family history also plays a role.

Many women with PCOS have difficulty using insulin, a hormone that facilitates the cells' use of glucose (energy) from the bloodstream. These women have too much insulin in their blood, provoking production of excessive androgens. High levels of androgens, such as testosterone, lead to acne, excessive hair growth (including facial hair), weight gain, and problems with ovulation that prevent pregnancy.

There is no cure for PCOS, so managing it is paramount to your health and to your chances of becoming pregnant. Treatment for PCOS should be tailored to your particular circumstances and should include a healthy diet and regular physical activity (with your doctor's approval).

Lifestyle plays a critical role in managing PCOS and promoting pregnancy. Many women with PCOS are overweight. If you weigh too much (see chapter 1 to find out), losing just 7 to 10 percent of your body weight—about twelve to eighteen pounds for a woman who weighs 175 pounds—can restore normal periods. Follow the MyPyramid Prepregnancy Eating Plan in chapter 3 to help you shed some pounds on a healthy diet. Include regular physical activity to naturally reduce blood glucose concentrations and make weight control easier. If you need more help, ask your doctor for a referral to an RD to help you develop the healthiest eating plan for your situation.

Metformin (found in Glucophage), a medication for treating type 2 diabetes, is useful in treating PCOS symptoms, too. Metformin helps to control blood glucose levels and reduce testosterone production. Another medication to stimulate ovulation, known as clomiphene citrate (found in Clomid and Serophane) may also be of use. A combination of metformin and clomiphene is helpful to some women. Surgery to bring on ovulation may also be the answer for some women to facilitate pregnancy.

If you suspect that you have PCOS, see your doctor for a complete physical exam. The following are symptoms of PCOS to consider:

- Family history—especially a mother or a sister with PCOS
- Infrequent menstrual periods, no menstrual periods, and/or irregular bleeding
- Insulin resistance or type 2 diabetes
- High cholesterol or high blood pressure
- Patches of thickened and dark brown or black skin on the neck, arms, breasts, or thighs
- Skin tags—tiny excess flaps of skin in the armpits or the neck area
- Pelvic pain
- Anxiety or depression
- An inability to become pregnant because of not ovulating
- Hirsutism—increased hair growth on the face, chest, stomach, back, thumbs, or toes—as well as male-pattern baldness or thinning hair
- Ovarian cysts
- Acne, oily skin, or dandruff
- Sleep apnea—excessive snoring and times when breathing stops during sleep

---

Trans Fat and Fertility

When you're trying to conceive, what you eat can matter as much as how much you eat. A recent study from the Harvard School of Public Health analyzed dietary habits and the ability to conceive in a group of more than eighteen thousand women with no history of infertility. The researchers found that the more trans fat there was in a woman's diet, the greater the likelihood of ovulatory infertility, such as PCOS. Eating a moderate amount of trans fat (2 percent of the total calories) amounted to a significantly lower conception rate among women in the group. On a 2,000-calorie diet, 2 percent of calories from trans fat amounts to about two tablespoons of stick margarine, one medium order of fast-food french fries, or one doughnut.

In a separate study, the Nurses' Health Study, Harvard researchers found that even when two diets contain the same amount of fat, the one that's higher in trans fat adds more pounds. Women who consumed 6 percent of their calories from trans fat (about 13 grams on a 2,000-calorie diet) were twelve pounds heavier after eight years than the women who consumed the same number of calories without any trans fat. See chapter 2 for more on trans fat.

Celiac Disease

In celiac disease, gluten—the protein found in wheat, barley, and rye—triggers an immune reaction in the body that damages the small intestine. The destruction that gluten causes reduces your capacity to absorb nutrients from foods. It may also be the reason for unexplained infertility in some women.

In 2003, the results of a large, multicenter study published in the *Archives of Internal Medicine* found celiac disease in 1 of every 133 Americans. Research also suggests a higher rate of celiac disease in women who are unable to become pregnant, and untreated celiac disease is associated with a higher miscarriage risk. Yet most people with celiac disease don't even know that they have it, mostly because it can be difficult to diagnose. Celiac disease is often misdiagnosed as irritable bowel syndrome. If you think you might have celiac disease, see a doctor for proper testing and a firm diagnosis. For more information about celiac disease, visit the Celiac Disease Foundation Web site, www.celiac.org. People with celiac disease should work closely with an RD who specializes in celiac disease to tailor an eating plan to fit their nutritional needs.

> ### WORDS OF
> *Motherly Wisdom*
>
> "When we went through fertility treatment, what helped me the most was when my doctor told me that it wasn't our fault that we were having difficulty getting pregnant. Eventually, I gave birth to healthy twin boys."
> —Lisa

Stress

For some couples, trying to get pregnant becomes stressful, especially as time passes. Women who have problems with fertility report higher levels of stress and anxiety than more fertile women do. Training yourself to feel calmer by using the relaxation response can be helpful when tension gets the better of you.

Here's how it works. The relaxation response lowers heart rate, blood pressure, and breathing rate, promoting relaxation. The best part is that those feelings of calm can remain for hours.

Deep breathing and meditation are two ways to elicit the relaxation response. *The Relaxation Response* and *Beyond the Relaxation Response*, both by Herbert Benson, M.D., provide instructions for eliciting the relaxation response. *Conquering Infertility: Dr. Alice Domar's Mind/Body Guide to Enhancing Fertility and Coping with Infertility* by Alice Domar, Ph.D., is an excellent resource for couples who are having trouble conceiving.

A balanced diet can help to relieve stress by providing the nutrients you need to stay energized. Limit your intake of caffeine and alcohol, to help to ensure that you get the rest you need at night so that you feel calmer during the day. Regular physical activity is also a great stress reliever.

From Here to Paternity: A Father's Preconception To-Do List

Prospective dads might think that their contribution to the next generation begins and ends at conception. In the past, the rest of the responsibility for making a baby was considered to be the woman's. That was mostly because the experts believed that only the fittest sperm could fertilize an egg. Now, however, we know that this is not the case. A pregnancy is affected by both of you, so before and after the positive pregnancy test, you and your partner should work together to live a healthy lifestyle, including eating right and exercising on a regular basis.

Here's what fathers-to-be should do before trying to make a baby:

Practice girth control. In a Danish study that included nearly sixteen hundred subjects, overweight men produced significantly less sperm. In addition to having higher sperm counts, the men in the normal-weight range—those with a BMI of 20 to 25—also had a lower percentage of abnormal sperm. A 2007 National Institutes of Health study found that the higher a man's BMI, the lower his fertility.

> WORDS OF
> *Motherly Wisdom*
>
> "We both needed to drop a few pounds, so my husband and I worked on weight control together before trying for a baby. Having a partner to work out with made it easier."
> —*Shana*

Take supplements. A balanced eating plan based on whole grains, fruits, vegetables, and low-fat protein foods helps to prevent a man from lacking the nutrients that are necessary for making top-notch sperm, particularly vitamin C, zinc, and folic acid. Although supplements are no substitute for a healthy diet, a daily multivitamin fills in small nutrient gaps that can sap fertility, so it is a good idea for men to take one (see chapter 3 to plan a healthy diet). The best multivitamin for men is one with very little or no iron that also provides about 100 percent of the Daily Value for the nutrients it contains. A man's daily iron requirement is less than half that of a woman's, so men typically satisfy their need for iron through food.

Evaluate medications. Certain drugs, including those for treating high blood pressure, ulcers, hair loss, and depression, can impair a man's ability to father a child. Check every medication with the pharmacist.

Get a move on. If your male partner is older than thirty, you might want to get going on baby making. The evidence is inconclusive, but it appears that his age affects his chances of getting a woman pregnant. One study of healthy nonsmokers found that fifty-year-old men made 20 percent less sperm than their thirty-year-old counterparts. The researchers estimate that sperm volume and mobility decrease by about 5 percent each year.

Stop smoking. If your male partner is still smoking, he should snuff the butts now. Smoking stresses sperm by creating free radicals that cause cell damage, by lowering sperm count, and by diminishing quality. A father's smoking habit can also increase his child's chances for leukemia and lymphoma, cancers of the blood.

Drop the drugs. Illegal drugs, including steroids, cocaine, and marijuana, can ruin the chances of conceiving. Marijuana renders sperm less fertile by turning them into hyperswimmers that burn out before they reach an egg. When you both smoke pot, your chances of conceiving are even less. Marijuana's active ingredient, THC, gets into a woman's reproductive organs and bodily fluids, and the sperm that are exposed to them become sluggish.

Cocaine may actually adhere to sperm without hampering its ability to fertilize the egg, increasing the chances of a child being affected by cocaine from the very moment of fertilization.

Limit alcohol use. Heavy drinkers produce sperm with defects that hinder their ability to fertilize an egg. Although the link between moderate drinking and fertility in men is murky, play it safe by limiting alcoholic beverages to no more than two drinks a day.

Shun chemicals. Take care with exposure to chemicals, especially at work. A man should make sure that his workplace provides proper protection and ventilation, especially if he is a painter, a janitor, or a printer or if he works in agriculture or in a laboratory.

Turn down the heat. Laptop computers can sabotage attempts at fatherhood, but only when they are perched on a man's lap. A study at the State University of New York at Stony Brook measured the scrotal temperatures of men who had been using laptop computers for sixty minutes. The researchers found that one hour of laptop use elevated scrotal temperature by about five degrees, enough to possibly impair sperm production. Men who prefer to use a laptop computer on their laps rather than on a desk or a table should invest in a laptop pad to keep the heat at bay.

Morning Sickness

Women who suffer from morning sickness will tell you that the nausea and vomiting associated with pregnancy can strike at any time of the day and anywhere: in public, in the car, and at work. Experts are unsure of the cause of the queasiness that's typically one of the first signs of pregnancy, but shifts in hormone levels are probably to blame. A heightened sense of smell perpetuated by hormonal surges often hinders any attempts to feel better, because offensive odors can easily trigger a wave of nausea or a bout of vomiting that wrecks your appetite.

Morning sickness seems to run the gamut: some women are queasy for a few weeks in the first trimester, and some mothers-to-be are sick on a daily basis until they deliver. For the most part, morning sickness ends early in the second trimester.

When you can't keep a bite of food or even just a few sips of water down, you are likely to wonder if your morning sickness is hurting the baby. In general, morning sickness is not harmful to your child unless it persists to the point where you're losing weight and becoming dehydrated. This is often the case with a condition called *hyperemesis gravidarum*, which affects tens of thousands of women every year. Women with hyperemesis gravidarum require medical supervision to ensure the body's proper balance and to monitor weight and conditions that jeopardize their health.

How do you know if your morning sickness is a cause for concern rather than a passing annoyance? According to the National Institutes of Health, the following are warning signals:

- A loss of two or more pounds
- Vomiting more than three times a day or the inability to keep food or liquid down
- Vomiting blood or material that resembles coffee grounds (call your health-care provider immediately)
- Nausea and vomiting that persist past your fourth month of pregnancy

If you're worried that your next pregnancy will be plagued by morning sickness as much as this one is, don't be. Each pregnancy is unique, and morning sickness with one baby does not predict the risk in future pregnancies. If it feels intolerable, try to keep in mind that morning sickness will disappear when your pregnancy ends.

The following tips can help you to better manage your morning sickness:

WORDS OF
Motherly Wisdom

"When I was pregnant with my first, the only things that made me feel better were cheese curls and lemonade. I ate them every day for the first few months."
—*Chris*

- Don't overdo it. Get plenty of sleep and relax whenever possible. Stress exacerbates the effects of morning sickness, which includes fatigue.
- Avoid rushing. Allow enough time to get out of bed in the morning and to get ready for the day. Some women leave crackers by the bed to munch on before they get up.
- Don't let yourself get too hungry. Dips in blood glucose levels can make matters worse. Eat small meals throughout the day and avoid fatty foods that aggravate your stomach.
- Eat what appeals to you, as long as it's considered safe during pregnancy. If that means soda and french fries for breakfast, so be it. Just remember to return to your MyPyramid plan as soon as you are able.

- Try eating more cold foods. Strong smells can trigger nausea; cold foods are less aromatic than warmer ones.
- Focus on carbohydrates. Plain baked potatoes, toast, rice, and pasta are easy on the stomach, and they're comforting, too.
- Take your prenatal vitamins at night, just before going to sleep, or with food, to reduce stomach irritation. Check with your health-care provider about switching from your prenatal vitamin to another type of multivitamin (such as chewables) until morning sickness passes.
- Consider acupressure wristbands, which are often employed to prevent seasickness. Look for them at pharmacies, marine specialty shops, and in health-food stores.
- Try acupuncture to relieve your distress. Look for an acupuncturist who is trained to work with pregnant women.
- Target and avoid your triggers. Offensive smells can set you off, affecting your appetite and the ability to keep food down. Limit your exposure to odors you find unpleasant by keeping rooms well ventilated and avoiding secondhand smoke.
- Sip ginger tea or flat ginger beer (this is not alcoholic beer). Ginger ale generally does not contain any real ginger. Peppermint tea is also soothing and is considered safe during pregnancy.
- Nibble on flavored popsicles for the fluid and the sugar.
- High doses of vitamin B_6—25 to 50 milligrams a day—can help to alleviate pregnancy-induced nausea. However, do not take large doses of vitamin B_6 or any other vitamin, dietary supplement, or medication without talking to your health-care provider first.

WORDS OF
Motherly Wisdom

"I couldn't be anywhere near meat or chicken when it was cooking. The smell of it was overwhelming and would make me sick."
—Diane

WORDS OF
Motherly Wisdom

"My nurse practitioner suggested sucking on lemon drops to relieve my nausea, and it really worked. I ate an entire bag at a hockey game once, just to avoid being sick in public."
—Jen

Gestational Diabetes

Your health-care provider should test your blood for gestational diabetes mellitus (GDM) between twenty-four and twenty-eight weeks of pregnancy. GDM is the form of diabetes that occurs for the first time when a woman is pregnant.

Having any type of diabetes means that the glucose (or sugar) level in your bloodstream is excessive, a condition called *hyperglycemia*. Glucose is the source of energy for every cell in your body and your baby's body.

In GDM, hyperglycemia happens because your body is unable to make and use all of the insulin it needs. Insulin helps glucose to enter the cells. When insulin does not do its job, there is a buildup of glucose in the blood. Although glucose is beneficial because it provides energy, too much is harmful to you and your baby.

Since your baby is receiving additional calories (in the form of glucose from your blood) on a steady basis, you could be carrying a large infant who has difficulty at delivery. Larger infants are prone to shoulder damage during delivery because it's harder for them to get through the birth canal. Mothers with GDM may need a cesarean section due to the baby's large size.

Children born to mothers with poorly controlled GDM are at greater risk for breathing problems, and they are more likely to become overweight in childhood or as adults. In addition, mothers with GDM may experience high blood pressure during pregnancy.

Are You at Risk?

GDM affects about 4 percent of all pregnancies—an estimated 135,000 cases each year in the United States. Experts aren't exactly sure why all cases of GDM happen, but there are definite risk factors, including having an immediate family member with diabetes, being overweight, having prediabetes, or having a history of GDM in a past pregnancy. Some groups—African Americans, Latinos, Native Americans, and Asian Americans/Pacific Islanders—are at greater risk for GDM, too.

Diagnosing GDM

The glucose challenge test is a reliable screening tool for GDM. For this test, you'll be asked to drink a sugary beverage. Then you will have your blood glucose tested one hour later. If it is not within the normal range, you will have to have another test, the oral glucose tolerance test (OGT), to confirm GDM. You have to fast for at least eight hours before the OGT test. The lab technician will take a baseline blood glucose level, then give you a sugary drink and test your glucose another three times: one hour, two hours, and three hours after you've finished the beverage. If your blood glucose concentration exceeds the normal level for two of the four readings, you have GDM.

Treating GDM

Once you find out that your GDM test is positive, every day counts for getting your blood glucose level under control. There is no need to panic, but you should immediately take steps to manage GDM with a balanced meal plan that's low in refined grains and added sugars. Ask your healthcare provider for a referral to an RD, who can help you to tailor a plan that works for you.

It takes work to manage GDM, but it's well worth the time and effort to ensure your and your baby's good health. You may need to increase your physical activity to help control your GDM. Working muscles gobble up glucose without your having to take glucose-lowering medication. You might also be asked to monitor your blood glucose concentration several times a day, and there's a possibility that you will need insulin injections to normalize your blood glucose level.

After the Baby Arrives

Gestational diabetes typically disappears once you've delivered. However, having GDM during one pregnancy puts you at greater risk for the condition in subsequent pregnancies. Some women with GDM develop type 2 diabetes later. You can prevent type 2 diabetes by achieving and maintaining a healthy weight and getting regular exercise after you deliver.

Ask your doctor about having a blood test six to twelve weeks after delivery to detect diabetes. To reduce your risk, get thirty minutes of physical activity on most days and follow a balanced eating plan. Women who have had gestational diabetes should continue to be tested for diabetes or prediabetes every one to two years.

Preterm Birth

Preterm birth—giving birth before thirty-seven weeks—is the most common obstetrical problem plaguing American women. About half a million women a year give birth too early.

Preterm delivery can happen to any woman, but some women are more prone to it than others. Although the cause of preterm birth is unidentifiable in about 50 percent of the cases, certain mothers-to-be are clearly at greater risk than others, including women who are expecting multiple babies, women who have had a preterm birth in the past, and women who have certain abnormalities of the uterus or cervix.

Health habits also influence the risk of preterm birth. Smoking cigarettes, using alcohol and drugs, domestic violence and other severe stress, a lack of social support, and standing for long periods are among them. Having diabetes, having elevated blood pressure, or weighing too much or too little before pregnancy all influence the risk of preterm birth, too.

Even if you have one or more risk factors for preterm birth, this does not mean that your baby will be born before your due date. However, you should take the best possible care of yourself and discuss with your doctor all of the ways you can prevent delivering early.

High Blood Pressure (Hypertension)

Some women enter pregnancy with chronic hypertension (high blood pressure), but more often, pregnancy provokes the condition. Hypertension is serious because it prevents the adequate flow of oxygen- and nutrient-rich blood to your baby by narrowing or constricting blood vessels in the uterus.

Blood pressure is the force of the blood pushing against the walls of your arteries, the vessels that transport blood to every part of the body, including to your developing baby. Using a blood pressure cuff and a stethoscope, your health-care provider will measure your blood pressure at every visit during your pregnancy.

Blood pressure readings consist of two numbers. The first, or top, number registers systolic pressure, the pressure in the arteries when your heart contracts. The second, or bottom, reading represents diastolic pressure, the pressure in the arteries when the heart relaxes between contractions. Normal blood pressure is below 120 over 80.

If your readings are consistently elevated at your regular prenatal visits, your health-care provider may suggest that you have your blood pressure taken on a regular basis in order to get a clearer picture. A diagnosis of hypertension prior to the twentieth week of pregnancy probably means that you have chronic hypertension—that your blood pressure won't revert to normal once you deliver.

Age, family history, and overall health have a bearing on the risk of pregnancy-induced hypertension (PIH). You're more prone to PIH if you:

- Are under twenty or older than thirty-five
- Had high blood pressure before conception
- Had diabetes before conception
- Have an immune disorder, including lupus
- Have kidney disease
- Have a history of drug or alcohol abuse or you smoke
- Have a family history of PIH
- Are underweight (BMI less than 19.8) or overweight (BMI of 26 or above)
- Are carrying more than one child

Managing your health to the best of your ability, eating a balanced diet, gaining the recommended number of pounds, and exercising regularly (if your doctor approves) are all ways to reduce the risk of PIH.

Preeclampsia

According to the March of Dimes, about 25 percent of women with chronic hypertension develop preeclampsia, a pregnancy complication that can come on quickly and is characterized by high blood pressure, swelling due to fluid retention, and abnormal kidney function that leads to protein in the urine. In addition to chronic hypertension, other risk factors for preeclampsia include being pregnant with more than one child, being overweight at conception and throughout pregnancy, having a history of preeclampsia, and being thirty-five or older, according to the American Dietetic Association.

An estimated 8 percent of women develop preeclampsia. It can show up at any point when you're expecting and immediately thereafter, but it typically occurs after the twentieth week of pregnancy. Swelling in the hands and feet, sudden weight gain, headaches, and changes in vision are indicators of preeclampsia; however, some women with a rapidly advancing form of the disease experience few symptoms. It's important to deal with preeclampsia immediately, because it is the primary cause of preterm delivery, serious illness, and maternal and fetal death.

The role of diet and dietary supplements in preventing preeclampsia is debatable. A 2007 review published in the *British Journal of Obstetrics and Gynaecology* suggests that calcium supplements might alleviate preeclampsia. The researchers, who pooled the results of twelve studies involving more than fifteen thousand women who took either 1,000 milligrams of calcium or a placebo (a sugar pill) each day, found that supplementation starting in early pregnancy reduced the incidence of high blood pressure and preeclampsia. The effect was greatest in women whose calcium consumption was low to begin with.

Other studies that used single nutrient dietary supplements, including vitamin C and vitamin E, have not shown promising results, however. According to a recent position paper by the American Dietetic Association, omega-3 fats (found in seafood, fortified foods, and dietary supplements) might prevent preeclampsia. The type of polyunsaturated fatty acids found in omega-3 fats, including DHA, counteracts elevated blood pressure. However, larger, long-term studies are necessary to truly determine the benefits.

An array of supplemental nutrients may be the key to holding preeclampsia at bay. Women who were of normal body weight before pregnancy and who used multivitamins at least once a week before conception and in the first three months of pregnancy reduced their risk of preeclampsia by 72 percent, compared to those who didn't take a multivitamin during this period, according to a study from the University of Pittsburgh Graduate School of Public Health. Research published in 2008 in the *American Journal of Obstetrics and Gynecology* found that taking multivitamin supplements that contain folic acid early in the second trimester and thereafter reduced preeclampsia in a group of nearly three thousand pregnant women. Both studies emphasize the importance of taking a daily multivitamin with folic acid during your childbearing years.

Weight gain between pregnancies poses a risk for preeclampsia in women who never had the condition, according to a 2007 report in *Obstetrics & Gynecology*. For now, it seems that the best approach to preventing preeclampsia is to enter pregnancy at a healthy weight and stick to the weight-gain guidelines provided in chapter 4, take a daily multivitamin pill prior to and throughout pregnancy, and eat a balanced diet that provides the nutrients you need, such as calcium, vitamins C and E, and healthy fats, including DHA.

Surviving Bed Rest

Most pregnant women get through pregnancy without major problems, but certain women—an estimated seven hundred thousand each year—find themselves on some form of bed rest to manage a variety of conditions, including preterm labor, inadequate or excessive amniotic fluid, high blood pressure, placenta previa (a condition in which the placenta implants on or near the cervix, increasing the risk of preterm birth), and poor fetal growth.

Bed rest varies. Some women are confined to rest only while they are at home. Others must stay in bed or on the couch all the time, getting up only to use the bathroom. Still other pregnant women are hospitalized to allow virtually no movement, with the goal of alleviating pressure on the cervix.

You may sometimes dream of just sitting and doing nothing, but when inactivity lasts for weeks or months, it gets old fast. All that lying down takes a toll on your physical health. Immobility weakens your muscles and wreaks havoc on your aerobic function. Moreover, by reducing your appetite, bed rest may encourage insufficient weight gain that could result in a low-birth-weight baby. Even when you're not particularly hungry, it's still important to stick with your pregnancy eating plan as much as possible; eat six or eight small meals a day instead of larger meals that may be more difficult to consume. Ask your doctor to recommend physical therapy for you while you're on bed rest. To find a physical therapist in your area, visit the American Physical Therapy Association's Web site, www.apta.org.

When you have other children or family responsibilities to fulfill, bed rest is a burden and wears on you quickly. Bed rest can be a financial yoke as well, because you are missing out on earning money and you might also need to hire someone to do the jobs you typically do, such as housecleaning and yard work.

You may be able to work from bed. If not, at least you can use your phone and your computer to communicate with the outside world and chat with others in the same situation. Groups such as Sidelines National Support Network (www.sidelines.org) offer support around the clock. Sidelines network chapters are staffed by volunteers who offer counseling, support, encouragement, and sometimes just a friendly ear to other women who are consigned to mandatory bed rest.

Dealing with Swelling

Swelling, or edema, is a normal, common part of pregnancy. It's due to a huge increase in the production of blood and other body fluids to meet the needs of your growing baby. You may have edema in your hands, face, legs, ankles, and feet. Pressure on your vena cava (the large vein on the right side of the body that is responsible for returning blood to your heart from your lower extremities) and on your pelvic veins make you prone to accumulating fluid in your legs, ankles, and feet.

You'll probably start experiencing edema when you reach your fifth month or so, although swelling can start at any point in your pregnancy. You may notice that your puffiness peaks at the end of the day.

A sudden change in fluid balance is a different matter; this may signal preeclampsia, which could endanger you and your baby. Call your healthcare provider immediately if you have sudden swelling. If your blood pressure and your urine are normal (they're checked at each prenatal visit), there is probably nothing to be concerned about.

Take the following steps to help diminish normal swelling:

- Avoid sitting or standing for long periods. It allows fluid to accumulate in your lower extremities.
- When you sit, elevate your feet.
- Engage in walking or swimming to move fluid out of the affected areas as much as possible. Water aerobics are helpful in reducing leg edema in pregnant women. Ask your doctor if this type of exercise is okay for you.

- Drink plenty of low-sodium fluids, such as water. Restricting fluid does not ease swelling, so drink up.
- Avoid processed and fast foods. Their high sodium content attracts water and helps your body to hold on to fluid. Focus on eating the recommended MyPyramid Plan servings of fresh fruits and vegetables; they are rich in potassium, a mineral that counteracts the effects of sodium.

Conclusion

You've just read about the many things that can go wrong in a pregnancy as well as the possible minor discomforts. When you're pregnant, you want it to go well, and the chances are good that it will. That's true even when complications such as diabetes or high blood pressure arise. Getting regular medical attention throughout your pregnancy, even when you feel fine, is the best way to ensure that you'll have the healthiest baby possible.

If you've read this book from cover to cover at this point, you've learned a lot about the most current thinking on how a healthy lifestyle affects your and your child's well-being. Your own experiences during pregnancy and parenthood will add to what you've discovered here.

This is not the end, however. There's still an entire chapter of delicious and nutritious recipes, followed by resources and scientific references for you to explore. The main part of this book has come to an end, but it's just the beginning of a lifetime with your new baby, and perhaps other family members to come. Enjoy it!

8

Quick and Delicious Recipes

The recipes in this chapter are full of good nutrition for you and your family. The dishes, drinks, and desserts are rich in the nutrients, such as protein, iron, and calcium, that you need to prepare for pregnancy, nourish a growing child, and feed your family. Most recipes call for lower-sodium and lower-fat versions of common ingredients, including chicken broth and dairy products, to help you adhere to the recommended limits for fat and sodium. There's no need to feel hemmed in, however. Go ahead and make the substitutions or additions that work best for you and your family. Enjoy!

Beverages

CAPPUCCINO
Makes 2 servings.

This drink can be a midmorning pick-me-up or a dessert. It is packed with bone-building calcium and protein.

1 cup 1% low-fat milk

2 teaspoons sugar

1 cup hot, strong, freshly brewed
  decaffeinated coffee or espresso

4 tablespoons fat-free whipped
  topping

Cinnamon or cocoa powder
  (optional)

In a small saucepan, heat the milk and sugar over medium heat until just hot. Place the hot milk mixture in a blender or a food processor. Blend on high speed until frothy (about 1 minute). Divide the hot coffee into two mugs, then pour half of the blended milk into each mug. Top with the whipped topping and sprinkle with cinnamon or cocoa powder, if desired.

Per Serving Calories: 108 • Total fat: 3 grams • Saturated fat: 2 grams • Trans fat: 0
Cholesterol: 11 milligrams • Sodium: 74 milligrams • Carbohydrate: 17 grams
Dietary fiber: 0 • Protein: 5 grams • Calcium: 180 milligrams • Iron: 0

LEMONADE
Makes 4 servings.

Homemade lemonade is better for you than store-bought because it contains more phytonutrients. Lemons help to calm morning sickness, too.

4 cups water

3 whole lemons

½ cup sugar

In a large saucepan, bring the water to a boil. Meanwhile, thinly slice the lemons. Add the sugar to the boiling water, stirring until it is dissolved. Pour the sugar-water mixture into a large heat-safe pitcher. Add the lemons and stir well. Refrigerate until chilled.

Per Serving Calories: 109 • Total fat: 0 • Saturated fat: 0 • Trans fat: 0 • Cholesterol: 0
Sodium: 1 milligram • Carbohydrate: 29 grams • Dietary fiber: 1 gram • Protein: 0
Calcium: 10 milligrams • Iron: 0

Mocha Java Smoothie

Makes 1 serving.

This drink is refreshing and filled with vitamin D, too.

1 teaspoon decaffeinated instant
  coffee granules

1 tablespoon warm water

1 cup 1% low-fat milk

2 tablespoons fat-free chocolate
  syrup

1 ice cube

In a small bowl, dissolve the coffee granules in the warm water, then place in a blender or a food processor. Add the milk, chocolate syrup, and ice cube. Blend on high speed for 1 to 2 minutes, or until frothy. Pour into a tall glass and drink immediately.

Per Serving Calories: 211 • Total fat: 3 grams • Saturated fat: 2 grams
Trans fat: n/a • Cholesterol: 12 milligrams • Sodium: 135 milligrams
Carbohydrate: 38 grams • Dietary fiber: 1 gram • Protein: 9 grams
Calcium: 300 milligrams • Iron: 1 milligram

Chocolate-Banana Blast

Makes 1 serving.

This calcium-rich beverage combines a serving of fruit and milk. Freeze the banana first for a frothier drink.

1 medium banana, peeled and
  sliced

1 cup 1% low-fat milk

2 tablespoons fat-free chocolate syrup

1 ice cube

Place the ingredients in a blender or a food processor. Blend on high speed for 1 to 2 minutes, or until frothy. Pour into a tall glass and drink immediately.

Per Serving Calories: 316 • Total fat: 3 grams • Saturated fat: 2 grams • Trans fat: n/a
Cholesterol: 12 milligrams • Sodium: 137 milligrams • Carbohydrate: 65 grams
Dietary fiber: 4 grams • Protein: 10 grams • Calcium: 300 milligrams
Iron: 1 milligram

BLUEBERRY-ORANGE SMOOTHIE
Makes 1 serving.

Are you in the mood for something fruity? This smoothie is sure to tempt your taste buds. Use fortified orange juice for even more vitamins and minerals.

1 cup fresh or frozen blueberries   ½ cup 100% orange juice
½ cup plain low-fat yogurt

Place the ingredients in a blender or a food processor. Blend on high speed for 1 to 2 minutes, or until frothy. Pour into a tall glass and drink immediately.

Per Serving Calories: 217 • Total fat: 3 grams • Saturated fat: 1 gram • Trans fat: n/a
Cholesterol: 7 milligrams • Sodium: 88 milligrams • Carbohydrate: 43 milligrams
Dietary fiber: 4 grams • Protein: 8 grams • Calcium: 250 milligrams • Iron: 1 milligram

CHERRY-BANANA COOLER
Makes 2 servings.

Fruit supplies natural sweetness plus beneficial fiber and phytonutrients. This smoothie supplies a hefty amount of fiber.

1 medium banana, peeled   ½ teaspoon vanilla extract
½ cup frozen or fresh sweet   Sugar or artificial sweetener
   cherries, pitted   (optional)
¾ cup plain low-fat yogurt   1 to 2 tablespoons milk (optional)

Place the banana in a blender or a food processor and process on high speed until smooth. Add the cherries, yogurt, vanilla extract, and sweetener, if desired. Process until well blended. Add milk for a thinner consistency. Pour into a tall glass and drink immediately.

Per Serving Calories: 182 • Total fat: 2 grams • Saturated fat: 1 gram • Trans fat: n/a
Cholesterol: 6 milligrams • Sodium: 65 milligrams • Carbohydrate: 38 grams
Dietary fiber: 4 grams • Protein: 6 grams • Calcium: 180 milligrams • Iron: 1 milligram

Soups and Stews

WHITE CHILI

Makes 8 servings.

Beans are bursting with antioxidants that thwart cell damage. Make a batch of this chili and freeze the leftovers.

1 tablespoon canola or olive oil

2 medium onions, peeled and chopped

3 cloves garlic, peeled and minced

3 15½-ounce cans great northern beans, drained and rinsed well

4 cups low-sodium chicken or vegetable broth

3 cups chopped cooked chicken

1 teaspoon ground cumin

½ teaspoon ground cloves

1 teaspoon dried oregano

2 cups shredded Monterey Jack cheese

In a large saucepan, heat the oil over medium heat. Add the onions and garlic and cook until the onions are translucent. Add the beans, broth, chicken, cumin, cloves, and oregano. Cover and simmer for about 1 hour. Remove from the heat and stir in the cheese until it melts.

Per Serving Calories: 373 • Total fat: 13 grams • Saturated fat: 6 grams • Trans fat: 0
Cholesterol: 61 milligrams • Sodium: 227 milligrams • Carbohydrate: 30 grams
Dietary fiber: 6 grams • Protein: 34 grams • Calcium: 300 milligrams • Iron: 4 milligrams

BEEF STEW

Makes 6 servings.

Serve this delicious dish spooned over mashed potatoes for a satisfying meal.

¼ cup all-purpose flour

½ teaspoon freshly ground black pepper

32 ounces boneless beef bottom round roast or other stew meat, cut into 1-inch pieces

1½ teaspoons crushed dried thyme leaves

1 teaspoon crushed dried basil leaves

2 14- or 14½-ounce cans reduced-sodium beef broth

5 teaspoons olive oil

Salt to taste

2 medium onions, peeled and chopped

6 cloves garlic, peeled and minced

12 ounces assorted small mushrooms

2 cups chopped fresh or frozen carrots

1 cup frozen peas

In a large bowl, combine the flour and black pepper. Add the meat and lightly coat it with the flour mixture. Set aside any remaining flour mixture.

In a stockpot, heat 2 teaspoons of the oil over medium heat until hot. Add half of the meat to the pan and brown, then remove the meat from the pan. Repeat with 1 teaspoon of the oil and the remaining meat. Remove the meat from the stockpot; season all of the meat with salt.

Heat the remaining 2 teaspoons of oil in the stockpot. Add the onions, garlic, thyme, and basil; cook and stir for 3 to 5 minutes. Add 1 can of beef broth and increase the heat to medium-high. Cook and stir for 1 to 2 minutes, or until the browned bits attached to the stockpot are dissolved. Stir in the remaining broth and any reserved flour mixture.

Return the meat to the stockpot. Stir in the mushrooms and bring to a boil. Reduce the heat, cover tightly, and simmer 1¼ hours. Add the carrots to the stockpot; continue simmering, covered, for 30 minutes or until the beef and carrots are fork-tender. Stir in the peas; simmer an additional 5 minutes.

Per Serving Calories: 361 • Total fat: 16 grams • Saturated fat: 5 grams • Trans fat: 0 Cholesterol: 87 milligrams • Sodium: 365 milligrams • Carbohydrate: 17 grams Dietary fiber: 3 grams • Protein: 36 grams • Calcium: 60 milligrams • Iron: 4 milligrams

---

CREAMY SWEET POTATO SOUP

Makes about 4 servings.

If you're short on time, use canned, drained sweet potatoes for this potassium- and calcium-packed soup.

2 tablespoons trans fat–free tub margarine

1 medium onion, peeled and diced

4 medium sweet potatoes, cooked, peeled, and chopped, or 4 cups cooked canned, drained, and chopped sweet potatoes

1 cup low-sodium chicken broth or stock

¼ teaspoon ground ginger

¼ teaspoon ground cumin

2 cups 2% reduced-fat milk or fortified soy beverage

In a medium saucepan, melt the margarine over medium heat. Add the onions and sauté until translucent. Transfer the onions to a blender or a food processor. Add the sweet potatoes, chicken broth or stock, ginger, and cumin. Puree until smooth. Return the mixture to the saucepan and add the milk or soy beverage. Warm gently. Serve immediately.

Note: Don't add the milk if you don't plan to eat all of the soup immediately. Take what you're going to eat of the sweet potato puree and add enough milk to achieve the desired consistency. Freeze the remaining sweet potato mixture or store it in the refrigerator for up to three days. Add the milk as you use it.

Per Serving Calories: 240 • Total fat: 9 grams • Saturated fat: 4 grams • Trans fat: 0
Cholesterol: 15 milligrams • Sodium: 158 milligrams • Carbohydrate: 33 grams
Dietary fiber: 4 grams • Protein: 8 grams • Calcium: 190 milligrams • Iron: 1 milligram

---

VEGGIE "STOUP"

Makes 6 servings.

This meal is not quite a soup and not quite a stew, but it's quite delicious and nutritious! Enjoy some now and freeze the rest for later.

2 tablespoons olive oil

½ cup diced carrots

3 stalks celery, diced

2 medium onions, peeled and diced

6 cloves garlic, peeled and minced

4 cups chopped zucchini

1 cup peeled and chopped eggplant

1 cup (or more) low-sodium chicken or vegetable broth or stock

1 28-ounce can whole tomatoes, undrained

1 10-ounce package fresh spinach, washed, with stems removed, and chopped

1 19-ounce can garbanzo beans, drained

2 teaspoons dried parsley

1 teaspoon dried thyme

1 teaspoon dried rosemary

Salt

Freshly ground black pepper

In a large soup pot, heat the oil over medium-high heat. Add the carrots, celery, onions, and garlic. Cook the vegetables until the onions are translucent. Add the zucchini and eggplant and cook for 5 to 7 minutes. Add the broth or stock and continue to cook for another 5 minutes. Add the tomatoes (with their juice), spinach, and garbanzo beans. Bring the mixture to a boil. Season with the parsley, thyme, rosemary, salt, and pepper.

For a thinner soup, use extra broth. As a stew, this can be served over cooked brown or white rice, whole-wheat or white cooked pasta, or whole-wheat couscous.

Per Serving Calories: 211 • Total fat: 6 grams • Saturated fat: 1 gram • Trans fat: 0
Cholesterol: 0 • Sodium: 335 milligrams • Carbohydrate: 34 grams
Dietary fiber: 7 grams • Protein: 9 grams • Calcium: 120 milligrams • Iron: 3 milligrams

---

Vegetables and Side Dishes

QUINOA SALAD

Makes 4 servings.

Quinoa, a grain that is rich in protein, iron, and fiber, provides a delicious alternative to rice.

2 cups low-sodium chicken or
 vegetable broth or stock
1 cup quinoa, uncooked
¾ cup chopped dried apricots
½ cup chopped pecans

¼ cup sliced scallions
2 tablespoons olive oil
3 tablespoons balsamic vinegar

In a medium saucepan, bring the broth or stock to a boil over high heat. Add the quinoa to the pan and cover. Reduce the heat to low and allow the quinoa to simmer for about 20 minutes, or until the liquid has been absorbed.

In a medium bowl, combine the apricots, pecans, and scallions and set aside.

In a small bowl, make the dressing by whisking the olive oil and vinegar until well blended. When the quinoa is done and has cooled, toss with the apricot-nut mixture and dressing. Chill for about 30 minutes before eating.

Per Serving Calories: 390 • Total fat: 20 grams • Saturated fat: 2 grams
Trans fat: n/a • Cholesterol: 0 • Sodium: 42 milligrams • Carbohydrate: 46 grams
Dietary fiber: 6 grams • Protein: 11 grams • Calcium: 50 milligrams • Iron: 3 milligrams

---

Carrot-Raisin Salad

Makes 4 servings.

This salad is easy to make, nutritious, and delicious!

2 cups grated carrots

½ cup raisins

2 tablespoons plain low-fat yogurt

2 tablespoons reduced-fat mayonnaise

In a medium bowl, combine the carrots and raisins. Add the yogurt and mayonnaise and toss well, coating the carrots and raisins.

Per Serving Calories: 89 • Total fat: 0 • Saturated fat: 0 • Trans fat: 0 Cholesterol: 0
Sodium: 46 milligrams • Carbohydrate: 22 grams • Dietary fiber: 2 grams
Protein: 2 grams • Calcium: 40 milligrams • Iron: 1 milligram

Broccoli-Rice Puff

Makes 8 servings.

Enjoy this dish on the side or have a larger serving as an entrée.

3 cups cooked wild rice or quick-cooking brown rice

4 cups cooked broccoli, chopped

2 tablespoons canola oil

2 cups chopped mushrooms

1 large onion, peeled and chopped

3 cloves garlic, peeled and chopped

½ teaspoon salt

½ teaspoon freshly ground black pepper

2 eggs, separated into yolks and whites

¾ cup fat-free half-and-half

1 cup shredded reduced-fat sharp cheddar cheese

Preheat the oven to 350°F.

Prepare a rectangular 3-quart baking dish by coating it with nonstick cooking spray.

In a large bowl, combine the rice and broccoli and set aside.

Heat the oil in a medium skillet. Add the mushrooms, onion, and garlic and cook over medium heat until the mushrooms are soft. Add the salt and pepper. Stir the mushroom mixture into the rice and broccoli mixture and blend well. Transfer the entire mixture to the baking dish.

In a small bowl, beat the egg yolks with the half-and-half for about 1 minute, using a whisk. Add the cheese (and more black pepper, if you like).

In another small bowl, beat the egg whites, using an electric mixer, until stiff but not dry (about 2 minutes). Fold the egg whites into the egg yolk mixture. Pour the egg mixture evenly over the rice and broccoli mixture. Bake for 25 minutes, or until the top is lightly browned.

Per Serving Calories: 153 • Total fat: 7 grams • Saturated fat: 1 gram • Trans fat: 0
Cholesterol: 107 milligrams • Sodium: 144 milligrams • Carbohydrate: 18 grams
Dietary fiber: 2 grams • Protein: 7 grams • Calcium: 40 milligrams • Iron: 1 milligram

---

TROPICAL SWEET POTATO MASH

Makes 2 servings.

This dish is a worthy partner for beef, chicken, or pork. It also makes a tasty snack or dessert when paired with a cup of vanilla yogurt.

1 medium sweet potato, cooked and peeled

1 tablespoon 100% orange juice

½ cup pineapple, crushed or chunks, drained

2 tablespoons chopped pecans or walnuts, roasted

Place the warm sweet potato and orange juice in a medium bowl and mash well. Stir in the pineapple. Place on a serving dish and sprinkle with the nuts.

Per Serving Calories: 286 • Total fat: 10 grams • Saturated fat: 1 gram • Trans fat: n/a
Cholesterol: 0 • Sodium: 42 milligrams • Carbohydrate: 43 milligrams
Dietary fiber: 6 grams • Protein: 4 grams • Calcium: 70 milligrams • Iron: 1 milligram

---

ROASTED VEGETABLE MEDLEY

Makes 4 servings.

Roasting brings out the natural flavors in vegetables.

1 pound new potatoes, washed and quartered

1 cup carrots, cut into 1-inch chunks

1 cup broccoli florets

1 cup cauliflower florets

2 small onions, peeled and cut into 4 wedges

¼ cup olive oil

3 cloves garlic, peeled and minced

1 teaspoon dried rosemary

1 teaspoon dried basil

Salt (optional)

Preheat the oven to 400°F. Place the vegetables in a large bowl and set aside.

In a small bowl, make the dressing by combining the olive oil, garlic, and dried herbs. Drizzle the mixture over the vegetables and stir well to fully coat.

Place the vegetable combination on an ungreased 9 × 13 inch baking sheet. Roast for about 20 minutes, or until the vegetables become fork-tender; toss after 10 minutes. Season with salt, if desired.

Per Serving (without added salt) Calories: 133 • Total fat: 1 gram • Saturated fat: 0
Trans fat: 0 • Cholesterol: 0 • Sodium: 44 milligrams • Carbohydrate: 27 grams
Dietary fiber: 5 grams • Protein: 4 grams • Calcium: 40 milligrams
Iron: 1 milligram

Mashed Potatoes with Spinach and Cheese

Makes 4 servings.

Evaporated milk supplies twice the calcium of regular milk in this healthier take on the classic comfort food.

1½ pounds Yukon Gold potatoes, washed and quartered

½ cup fat-free evaporated milk

2 tablespoons low-fat sour cream

¾ cup shredded sharp reduced-fat cheddar cheese

2 cups baby spinach leaves, washed and shredded

Freshly ground black pepper

In a medium saucepan, boil the potatoes for 15 to 20 minutes, or until tender. Drain well and return to the pan. Add the evaporated milk and sour cream. Beat the potato mixture with an electric mixer on low speed until it is light and fluffy, or mash by hand. Transfer the mixture to a serving bowl. Add the cheese, spinach, and pepper and stir. Serve warm.

Per Serving Calories: 211 • Total fat: 3 grams • Saturated fat: 2 grams • Trans fat: n/a
Cholesterol: 10 milligrams • Sodium: 213 milligrams • Carbohydrate: 36 grams
Dietary fiber: 4 grams • Protein: 12 grams • Calcium: 240 milligrams • Iron: 2 milligrams

Entrées

CHICKEN AND COUSCOUS
Makes 2 servings.

Use whole-wheat couscous instead of white to work in more fiber, vitamins, and minerals.

1½ cups low-sodium chicken broth or stock

½ cup couscous, uncooked

2 teaspoons olive oil

1 small onion, peeled and sliced thin

8 ounces boneless, skinless chicken breasts, cut in ½-inch cubes

2 cloves garlic, peeled and diced

¼ teaspoon ground cumin

¼ teaspoon ground ginger

¼ teaspoon ground cinnamon

1 cup grated carrots

½ cup dried cranberries

¼ cup slivered almonds

In a small saucepan, bring 1 cup of the broth or stock to a boil. Add the couscous. Cover, turn off the heat, and let stand for 5 minutes.

In a large skillet, heat the oil over medium-high heat. Add the onion and sauté until translucent, about 3 minutes. Add the chicken and brown. Add the remaining ½ cup of broth or stock as well as the garlic, cumin, ginger, and cinnamon. Let simmer until the meat is cooked through, 5 to 7 minutes.

Place the cooked couscous in a large serving bowl. Add the chicken mixture and stir. Add the carrots and cranberries and mix well. Garnish with the almonds just before serving.

Per Serving Calories: 455 • Total fat: 15 grams • Saturated fat: 2 grams
Trans fat: 0 • Cholesterol: 0 • Sodium: 98 milligrams • Carbohydrate: 68 grams
Dietary fiber: 7 grams • Protein: 14 grams • Calcium: 90 milligrams
Iron: 2 milligrams

BROCCOLI AND CHEDDAR QUICHE
Makes 6 servings.

Evaporated milk is mostly responsible for this quiche's whopping 960 milligrams of calcium per serving—nearly a day's worth.

2 tablespoons trans fat–free
   tub margarine
1 medium onion, peeled and
   chopped
1 12-ounce can 2% evaporated
   milk
2 whole eggs
2 egg whites

¼ cup all-purpose flour
¼ teaspoon freshly ground
   black pepper
1 cup reduced-fat shredded
   cheddar cheese
1 10-ounce box chopped frozen
   broccoli, thawed, or 2 cups fresh
   broccoli, cooked and chopped

Preheat the oven to 350°F. Lightly coat a 10-inch pie pan with vegetable cooking spray.

In a medium skillet, heat the margarine over medium heat. Add the onions and sauté until translucent. Set aside.

In a medium bowl, whisk together the evaporated milk, whole eggs, egg whites, flour, and pepper. Set aside.

Sprinkle ½ cup of the cheese into the pie pan. Top with the cooked onions and the broccoli.

Pour the milk and egg mixture into the pie pan. Sprinkle with the remaining cheese.

Bake for 35 to 40 minutes, or until a knife inserted in the center comes out clean. Cool on a wire rack for 10 minutes before serving.

Per Serving Calories: 395 • Total fat: 11 grams • Saturated fat: 5 grams • Trans fat: 0
Cholesterol: 148 milligrams • Sodium: 556 milligrams • Carbohydrate: 42 grams
Dietary fiber: 2 grams • Protein: 32 grams • Calcium: 960 milligrams • Iron: 2 milligrams

---

SHRIMP AND ASPARAGUS STIR-FRY

Makes 2 servings.

Cooked shrimp saves time when you're preparing this protein-packed dish.

1 teaspoon canola oil
½ medium onion, peeled and
   chopped
½ cup chopped red bell pepper
½ cup chopped green bell pepper
2 cloves garlic, peeled and minced
1 cup raw asparagus,
   chopped into 1-inch lengths

8 ounces frozen cooked shrimp,
   defrosted
1 tablespoon reduced-sodium
   soy sauce
½ cup canned pineapple chunks,
   drained

In a large skillet, heat the oil over high heat. Add the onions, peppers, garlic, and asparagus. Stir-fry for about 5 minutes, or until the vegetables are slightly browned. Add the shrimp and soy sauce to the pan. Cook for an additional 3 minutes. Add the pineapple and stir. Serve over cooked white or brown rice.

Per Serving Calories: 261 • Total fat: 9 grams • Saturated fat: 1 gram • Trans fat: 0
Cholesterol: 170 milligrams • Sodium: 472 milligrams • Carbohydrate: 19 grams
Dietary fiber: 4 grams • Protein: 26 grams • Calcium: 100 milligrams
Iron: 5 milligrams

EASY ROASTED PORK LOIN

Makes 3 servings.

Surprise! Pork tenderloin has even less fat than boneless, skinless, chicken breast.

2 cloves garlic, peeled and crushed

1 teaspoon dried rosemary

2 tablespoons olive oil

2 tablespoons balsamic vinegar

¼ teaspoon salt

¼ teaspoon freshly
  ground black pepper

1 pork tenderloin (about
  ¾ pound)

1 medium onion, peeled and
  quartered

1 cup baby carrots

Preheat the oven to 400°F.

In a small bowl, combine the garlic, rosemary, olive oil, balsamic vinegar, salt, and pepper. Place the pork, onions, and carrots in a baking dish. Pour the olive oil and balsamic vinegar mixture into the baking dish, tossing to coat the vegetables and the meat.

Bake for about 20 minutes, or until a meat thermometer registers that the internal temperature is 160°F.

Per Serving Calories: 186 • Total fat: 7 grams • Saturated fat: 3 grams • Trans fat: 0
Cholesterol: 54 milligrams • Sodium: 488 milligrams • Carbohydrate: 6 grams
Dietary fiber: 2 grams • Protein: 24 grams • Calcium: 20 milligrams
Iron: 1 milligram

BARBEQUE PORK SKILLET[*]

Makes 4 servings.

This tasty dish is quick to make.

1 teaspoon canola oil

4 pork chops, ¾-inch thick

¼ cup Italian dressing

¼ cup barbecue sauce

In a large skillet, heat the oil over medium-high heat. Brown the chops for about 1 minute on each side.

Add the dressing and barbecue sauce to the pan, stirring to blend. Cover and simmer for 5 to 8 minutes.

Per Serving Calories: 180 • Total fat: 7 grams • Saturated fat: 3 grams • Trans fat: 0
Cholesterol: 60 milligrams • Sodium: 430 milligrams • Carbohydrate: 3 grams
Dietary fiber: 0 • Protein: 25 grams • Calcium: 11 milligrams • Iron: 1 milligram

---

[*]This recipe is used with permission of the National Pork Board.

STUFFED PEPPERS

Makes 6 servings.

Green peppers are rich in vitamin C. Use wild or brown rice to work in a whole grain.

6 large green bell peppers, cut in half lengthwise and cleaned of stems, seeds, and membranes

1 medium onion, peeled and chopped

1 teaspoon olive oil

2 cups cooked rice

1 14½-ounce can no-salt-added stewed tomatoes, undrained

2 tablespoons tomato paste

1 tablespoon dried basil

1 cup low-fat, low-sodium cottage cheese

¾ cup shredded reduced-fat cheddar cheese

Preheat the oven to 350°F.

In a large saucepan, boil the peppers for 3 to 5 minutes. Remove with a slotted spoon, drain the excess water, and return to the pan.

In a small nonstick skillet, sauté the onions in the oil until translucent.

Transfer the onions to a large bowl. Add the rice, tomatoes with their juice, tomato paste, basil, and cottage cheese and stir to combine. Place the peppers in a 9 × 13 inch baking dish. Spoon the cottage cheese and rice mixture into the pepper shells, dividing evenly. Top each pepper with an equal amount of cheddar cheese. Bake for 25 minutes, or until heated through.

Per Serving Calories: 179 • Total fat: 2 grams • Saturated fat: 1 gram • Trans fat: n/a
Cholesterol: 5 milligrams • Sodium: 296 milligrams • Carbohydrate: 29 grams
Dietary fiber: 4 grams • Protein: 13 grams • Calcium: 140 milligrams • Iron: 3 milligrams

---

SPAGHETTI WITH SHRIMP, SPINACH, AND TOMATOES

Makes 4 servings.

This colorful, iron-rich dish includes foods from MyPyramid's meat, vegetable, and grain groups.

8 ounces whole-wheat spaghetti, uncooked

¼ cup olive oil

1 onion, peeled and diced

3 cloves garlic, peeled and minced

1 pound large raw shrimp, peeled and cleaned, or frozen cooked shrimp, defrosted

4 cups baby spinach, washed and dried

20 cherry tomatoes, cut in half

Salt (optional)

Freshly ground black pepper (optional)

Cook the spaghetti according to the package directions. Drain well and set aside.

In a large skillet, heat 2 tablespoons of the olive oil over medium heat. Add the onion and garlic; sauté for about 3 minutes, or until just tender. Add the shrimp to the pan and cook for 3 minutes. (If you're using cooked shrimp, add them to the pan after cooking the onion, garlic, spinach and tomatoes. Toss the shrimp until they are warm, about 3 minutes.) Stir in the spinach and tomatoes and continue to cook until the shrimp are cooked through and the spinach and tomatoes are soft, about 4 minutes. Toss the cooked, drained pasta with the shrimp mixture and the remaining olive oil. Season with salt and pepper, if desired.

Per Serving Calories: 437 • Total fat: 11 grams • Saturated fat: 2 grams • Trans fat: n/a
Cholesterol: 113 milligrams • Sodium: 128 milligrams • Carbohydrate: 61 grams
Dietary fiber: 7 grams • Protein: 27 grams • Calcium: 90 milligrams • Iron: 5 milligrams

---

Fettuccine with Mushrooms and Prosciutto

Makes 4 servings.

This elegant entrée only sounds time-consuming. Whip up a batch tonight and enjoy some for lunch tomorrow.

16 ounces spinach fettuccine, uncooked

2 tablespoons olive oil

8 ounces sliced white mushrooms

½ cup light cream

½ cup fat-free half-and-half

¼ pound prosciutto (or ham), cut into thin strips

¼ cup grated Parmesan cheese

Cook the fettuccine according to the package directions. Drain well and set aside.

In a large skillet, heat the oil over medium-high heat. Add the mushrooms and sauté until soft, about 10 minutes. Stir in the cream, half-and-half, and prosciutto. Bring to a simmer. Add the cheese and stir. Toss the cooked, drained pasta with the sauce in the pan. Serve warm.

Per Serving Calories: 628 • Total fat: 17 grams • Saturated fat: 6 grams • Trans fat: 0
Cholesterol: 39 milligrams • Sodium: 489 milligrams • Carbohydrate: 91 grams
Dietary fiber: 13 grams • Protein: 26 grams • Calcium: 190 milligrams • Iron: 3 milligrams

---

Cold Satay Noodle Salad

Makes 2 servings.

To make this dish meatless, substitute tofu for the chicken.

8 ounces whole-wheat spaghetti, uncooked

¼ cup peanut butter or sunflower nut butter

1 tablespoon honey

2 tablespoons warm water

1 tablespoon reduced-sodium soy sauce

2 tablespoons lime juice

1 tablespoon canola oil

8 ounces cooked, boneless skinless chicken, chopped

1 cup fresh baby spinach, washed and dried

½ cup grated carrots

2 scallions, thinly sliced at an angle

2 tablespoons chopped peanuts or sunflower seeds

1 tablespoon chopped fresh cilantro (optional)

Cook the spaghetti according to the package directions. Drain well and set aside.

In a large bowl, combine the peanut butter, honey, and warm water. Add the soy sauce and lime juice. Using a whisk, add the canola oil. Add the cooked, drained spaghetti and toss well to coat. Add the chicken, spinach, carrots, and scallions and toss well. Place the noodle mixture on a serving dish and garnish with the nuts or seeds and the cilantro, if desired.

Per Serving Calories: 431 • Total fat: 15 grams • Saturated fat: 3 grams
Trans fat: 0 • Cholesterol: 32 milligrams • Sodium: 310 milligrams
Carbohydrate: 53 milligrams • Dietary fiber: 7 grams • Protein: 27 grams
Calcium: 60 milligrams • Iron: 3 milligrams

ZITI WITH RED PEPPER SAUCE

Makes 4 servings.

*This recipe is meatless, but there is no shortage of protein
in this attractive entrée.*

8 ounces ziti or rotini, uncooked

2 teaspoons olive oil

1 medium onion, peeled and chopped

¾ cups low-sodium chicken broth

1 cup low-fat, low-sodium cottage cheese

1 19-ounce jar roasted red peppers, drained and well rinsed

½ teaspoon dried thyme

¼ teaspoon salt

2 cups broccoli, chopped and cooked (thawed frozen broccoli can be used)

Freshly ground black pepper

Cook the ziti according to the package directions. Drain well and set aside.

In a large nonstick skillet, heat the oil over medium heat. Add the onions and sauté until translucent. Add the chicken broth and continue to simmer for about 3 minutes.

Place the cottage cheese in a food processor and blend until smooth. Add the red peppers, thyme, and salt and blend for another minute, adding some chicken broth, if necessary, to achieve the desired consistency.

Transfer the red pepper and cottage cheese mixture to the skillet and heat gently, stirring often, for about 3 minutes. Add the broccoli and the cooked, drained pasta, season with pepper, and toss well. Serve warm.

Per Serving Calories: 323 • Total fat: 4 grams • Saturated fat: 1 gram • Trans fat: 0
Cholesterol: 2 milligrams • Sodium: 203 milligrams • Carbohydrate: 54 grams
Dietary fiber: 5 grams • Protein: 18 grams • Calcium: 90 milligrams
Iron: 3 milligrams

ALL-GROWN-UP MAC AND CHEESE
Makes 6 servings.

This sophisticated version of a children's favorite will please the entire family. Use whole-wheat pasta, if you like.

8 ounces elbow macaroni, uncooked

2 tablespoons trans fat–free tub margarine

2 medium onions, peeled and chopped

2 cups shredded reduced-fat sharp cheddar cheese

1 tablespoon dried parsley

½ teaspoon freshly ground black pepper

2 cups low-fat, low-sodium cottage cheese

½ cup 1% low-fat milk

¼ cup seasoned bread crumbs

¼ cup shredded Parmesan cheese

Preheat the oven to 350°F. Spray a 2-quart baking dish with nonstick cooking spray and set aside.

Cook the macaroni according to the package directions. Drain well and set aside.

In a small skillet, heat the margarine over medium heat. Add the onions and sauté until translucent. Set aside.

In a large bowl, combine the cooked, drained macaroni, onions, cheddar cheese, parsley, and pepper. Set aside.

Place the cottage cheese and milk in a food processor or a blender. Blend until smooth. Pour this mixture into the bowl with the macaroni and mix well. Pour the entire mixture into the baking dish.

In a small bowl, combine the bread crumbs and Parmesan cheese. Sprinkle over the top of the macaroni mixture. Bake for about 30 minutes, or until hot in the center.

Per Serving Calories: 346 • Total fat: 9 grams • Saturated fat: 4 grams • Trans fat: 0
Cholesterol: 16 milligrams • Sodium: 435 milligrams • Carbohydrate: 39 grams
Dietary fiber: 2 grams • Protein: 27 grams • Calcium: 300 milligrams • Iron: 2 milligrams

---

TURKEY POTPIE

Makes 6 servings.

Nothing says comfort like a potpie. This one is far lower in fat and higher in nutrients than the store-bought versions.

Filling

2 cups fresh or frozen chopped carrots

½ cup low-sodium chicken or vegetable broth

1½ cups 1% low-fat milk

⅓ cup all-purpose flour

1 teaspoon dried sage leaves, crushed

1 tablespoon trans fat–free tub margarine

¼ teaspoon salt

2 cups cooked turkey, cut into ½-inch cubes

1 cup fresh or frozen peas

Topping

1 cup all-purpose flour

1 teaspoon baking powder

¼ teaspoon salt

⅛ teaspoon baking soda

2 tablespoons trans fat–free tub margarine

½ cup fat-free buttermilk

Preheat the oven to 400°F. Spray a 2-quart baking dish with nonstick cooking spray and set aside.

In a large saucepan, combine the carrots and broth and bring to a boil. Cover and reduce the heat, simmering for 2 to 3 minutes, or until the carrots are crisp-tender.

In a small bowl, whisk together the milk and flour and blend well. Stir the milk mixture, sage, margarine, and salt into the carrot mixture. Bring to a boil, stirring constantly, then boil for 1 minute longer. Stir in the turkey and peas. Pour the entire filling mixture into the baking dish and set aside while you make the topping.

In a medium bowl, combine the flour, baking powder, salt, and baking soda and stir. Cut in the margarine until the mixture resembles coarse meal. Add the buttermilk, stirring well to mix. Drop by teaspoonfuls onto the turkey mixture, covering it entirely. Bake for 25 to 30 minutes, or until the topping is golden brown.

Per Serving Calories: 273 • Total fat: 8 grams • Saturated fat: 2 grams
Trans fat: 0 • Cholesterol: 36 milligrams • Sodium: 365 milligrams
Carbohydrate: 30 grams • Dietary fiber: 2 grams • Protein: 21 grams
Calcium: 170 milligrams • Iron: 2 milligrams

TACO SALAD

Makes 1 serving.

Black beans and corn lend fiber, phytonutrients, and protein to this nutritious and delicious main-dish salad.

2 cups leafy greens, such as romaine lettuce

1 medium tomato, chopped

Quarter of an avocado, peeled and sliced

½ cup canned black beans, drained and rinsed well

½ cup cooked corn

½ cup crumbled baked tortilla chips

¼ cup shredded reduced-fat cheddar cheese

1 teaspoon olive oil

1 tablespoon lime juice

Fresh cilantro, chopped (optional)

In a medium bowl, toss together the greens, tomato, avocado, beans, and corn. Toss with the tortilla chips and cheese. Dress with the olive oil and lime juice. Transfer to a plate and garnish with cilantro, if desired.

Per Serving Calories: 484 • Total fat: 13 grams • Saturated fat: 3 grams
Trans fat: n/a • Cholesterol: 8 milligrams • Sodium: 749 milligrams
Carbohydrate: 72 grams • Dietary fiber: 15 grams • Protein: 23 grams
Calcium: 260 milligrams • Iron: 4 milligrams

SHEPHERD'S PIE

Makes 8 servings.

This is a real-crowd pleaser, especially on a cold night. Add a simple green salad, and you've got yourself a meal.

6 medium Yukon Gold potatoes

8 ounces ground beef, at least 90% lean

8 ounces 100% lean ground turkey or chicken breast meat

1 10¾-ounce can reduced-sodium condensed tomato soup

1 14½-ounce can diced tomatoes with green pepper, celery, and onion, drained

2 14½-ounce cans no-salt-added green beans, drained

1 15¼-ounce can no-salt-added corn, drained

2 tablespoons trans fat–free tub margarine

1 5-ounce can low-fat evaporated milk

1 cup shredded reduced-fat cheddar cheese

Preheat the oven to 350°F. Peel the potatoes and chop into 1-inch chunks. Place in a medium saucepan and cover with water. Boil over medium-high heat until soft. When they are done, drain them well, return them to the pan, cover, and set aside.

In a medium skillet coated with nonstick cooking spray, brown the ground beef and ground turkey over medium-high heat, breaking up the large pieces, until no longer pink—about 5 minutes. Drain well and place in an ungreased 9 × 13 inch baking dish. Add the tomato soup, tomatoes, green beans, and corn to the meat. Mix well.

Mash the margarine and evaporated milk into the potatoes. Spread the mashed potatoes evenly on top of the meat and vegetable mixture. Top with the cheese.

Bake for 20 to 25 minutes, or until hot. Cool for 5 to 10 minutes before serving.

Per Serving Calories: 384 • Total fat: 8 grams • Saturated fat: 3 grams • Trans fat: 0
Cholesterol: 37 milligrams • Sodium: 531 milligrams • Carbohydrate: 58 grams
Dietary fiber: 8 grams • Protein: 24 grams • Calcium: 160 milligrams
Iron: 4 milligrams

HASH BROWN SCRAMBLE

Makes 4 servings.

Eggs are one of the only natural food sources of vitamin D.

1 tablespoon canola or olive oil

2 cups refrigerated or frozen
hash brown potatoes, thawed

¼ cup sliced mushrooms

1 small onion, peeled and chopped

½ cup chopped red bell pepper

4 eggs

¼ cup 1% low-fat milk

½ teaspoon salt

¼ teaspoon freshly ground pepper

In a medium skillet, heat the oil over medium heat. Add the hash browns and cook for a few minutes until heated through, stirring occasionally. Add the mushrooms, onions, and bell pepper. Sauté for 6 or 7 minutes, stirring constantly.

In a medium bowl, whisk together the eggs and milk. Add the salt and pepper and stir to combine. Pour the mixture evenly over the vegetables in the skillet. As mixture begins to set, gently draw an inverted pancake turner completely across the bottom and the sides of the pan so that the egg cooks, forming large, soft curds. Continue cooking until the eggs are thickened and no visible liquid egg remains.

Per Serving Calories: 210 • Total fat: 9 grams • Saturated fat: 2 grams • Trans fat: 0
Cholesterol: 212 milligrams • Sodium: 390 milligrams • Carbohydrate: 23 grams
Dietary fiber: 2 grams • Protein: 10 grams • Calcium: 60 milligrams • Iron: 1 milligram

WALNUT-CHICKEN STIR FRY

Makes 4 servings.

Walnuts contain heart-healthy fats, and ginger quells a queasy stomach.

2 tablespoons tomato paste

2 tablespoons low-sodium tomato
juice

2 tablespoons reduced-sodium soy
sauce

¼ cup chopped walnuts

½ cup chopped red bell pepper

½ cup snow peas

½ cup chopped onion

2 teaspoons cornstarch

2 teaspoons toasted sesame oil

2 tablespoons freshly grated
(peeled) ginger root

16 ounces boneless, skinless
chicken breast meat, cut into
½-inch cubes

2 tablespoons water or chicken
broth

Freshly ground black pepper
(optional)

In a large bowl, use a whisk to combine the tomato paste, tomato juice, soy sauce, cornstarch, sesame oil, and ginger. Add the chicken and toss to coat the meat. Set aside.

Coat a wok or a large nonstick skillet with nonstick cooking spray and place over moderate heat. When the wok is hot, add the chicken mixture and stir constantly for 2 minutes. Add the walnuts, bell pepper, snow peas, onions, and water and stir constantly for 2 more minutes, or until the chicken is cooked through. Season with pepper, if desired. Transfer to a serving platter. Serve with cooked white or brown rice.

Per Serving Calories: 296 • Total fat: 10 grams • Saturated fat: 1 gram • Trans fat: 0
Cholesterol: 65 milligrams • Sodium: 442 milligrams • Carbohydrate: 21 grams
Dietary fiber: 2 grams • Protein: 28 grams • Calcium: 40 milligrams • Iron: 2 milligrams

HONEY-ORANGE SALMON FILLET

Makes 2 servings.

Salmon supplies DHA, a beneficial omega-3 fat for your baby's brain and vision and your general well-being. Serve with steamed asparagus or green beans and whole-wheat couscous for a balanced meal.

¼ cup honey

½ cup 100% orange juice

2 tablespoons reduced-sodium soy
sauce

2 cloves garlic, peeled and thinly
sliced

2 tablespoons thinly sliced scallions

1 tablespoon thinly sliced (peeled)
fresh ginger

½ teaspoon freshly ground black
pepper

8 ounces salmon fillet

In a small bowl, mix the honey, orange juice, soy sauce, garlic, scallions, ginger, and black pepper. Place the salmon skin side up in a shallow dish and coat with the marinade. Cover and marinate in the refrigerator for 30 minutes.

Spray a medium skillet with nonstick cooking spray. Place the salmon skin side down in the pan, along with the remaining marinade. Cover and simmer over medium heat until the salmon is cooked through, 15 to 20 minutes.

Per Serving Calories: 373 • Total fat: 12 grams • Saturated fat: 2 grams • Trans fat: 0
Cholesterol: 66 milligrams • Sodium: 669 milligrams • Carbohydrate: 43 grams
Dietary fiber: 1 gram • Protein: 24 grams • Calcium: 30 milligrams • Iron: 1 milligram

HALIBUT WITH CREAMY DIJON SAUCE
Makes 4 servings.

Halibut harbors a host of nutrients, including magnesium, iodine, vitamin B_6, and potassium, that you and your baby need.

1 tablespoon trans fat–free tub margarine, melted

½ teaspoon onion powder

¼ teaspoon dried marjoram

¼ teaspoon plus ⅛ teaspoon dried thyme

1½ pounds halibut, about 1 inch thick

½ cup low-fat sour cream

1 tablespoon all-purpose flour

1 tablespoon Dijon-style mustard

¼ teaspoon freshly ground black pepper

½ cup low-sodium chicken or vegetable broth

Preheat the oven broiler. In a small bowl, combine the margarine, onion powder, marjoram, and ¼ teaspoon thyme. Place the fish on the rack of an unheated broiler pan. Brush the fish with the margarine mixture. Broil for 5 minutes, turn, brush with the remaining sauce, and broil for 3 to 7 minutes more, or until the fish flakes easily with a fork.

In a small saucepan, stir together the sour cream, flour, mustard, black pepper, and ⅛ teaspoon thyme. Add the broth and stir until well mixed. Cook and stir over medium heat until the mixture is thickened and bubbly, then cook and stir for 1 more minute. To serve, top the fish with the Dijon sauce.

Per Serving Calories: 233 • Total fat: 8 grams • Saturated fat: 3 grams • Trans fat: 0
Cholesterol: 66 milligrams • Sodium: 155 milligrams • Carbohydrate: 2 grams
Dietary fiber: 0 • Protein: 37 grams • Calcium: 110 milligrams • Iron: 2 milligrams

Sandwiches, Burgers, and Pizza

BEEF POCKETS

Makes 4 servings.

*This recipe covers a lot of ground by including foods from
MyPyramid's meat, vegetable, grain, and milk groups.*

1 pound ground beef, at least 90%
lean (or textured vegetable protein
crumbles)

1 tablespoon chili powder (optional)

1 10-ounce package frozen chopped
spinach, thawed and well drained

½ cup salsa, plus extra for optional
garnish

4 medium whole-wheat pita breads,
sliced in half

½ cup shredded reduced-fat
cheddar cheese

In a medium skillet, brown the ground beef over medium heat until it's
no longer pink. Pour off the drippings. Season the beef with the chili
powder, if desired. Stir in the spinach and salsa. Cook over medium
heat until heated through. To serve, place the beef and vegetable
mixture in the pita pockets along with equal amounts of cheese (and
more salsa, if desired).

Per Serving (2 pockets) Calories: 425 • Total fat: 14 grams
Saturated fat: 6 grams • Trans fat: 1 gram • Cholesterol: 76 milligrams
Sodium: 762 milligrams • Carbohydrate: 41 grams • Dietary fiber: 7 grams
Protein: 36 grams • Calcium: 190 milligrams • Iron: 6 milligrams

---

BLACK BEAN AND CHEESE QUESADILLAS

Makes 2 servings.

*This is so easy yet so good for you, too! Serve with a simple
green salad or fruit.*

4 7-inch whole-wheat tortillas

¾ cup shredded reduced-fat
Monterey Jack cheese

¾ cup canned black beans, rinsed

¼ cup diced red bell pepper

Salsa (optional)

Low-fat sour cream (optional)

Coat a medium skillet or a griddle with nonstick cooking spray. Over low heat, add 1 of the tortillas (or 2, if you're working on a griddle) and top (each) with a quarter of the cheese, beans, and bell pepper. Cover (each) with another tortilla. Cook about 2 minutes on each side, gently pressing down on the quesadilla to melt the cheese. Serve with salsa and sour cream, if desired.

Per Serving (without the salsa and sour cream) Calories: 429 • Total fat: 6 grams
Saturated fat: 3 grams • Trans fat: n/a • Cholesterol: 10 millgrams
Sodium: 967 milligrams • Carbohydrate: 70 milligrams • Dietary fiber: 13 grams
Protein: 25 grams • Calcium: 240 milligrams • Iron: 5 milligrams

Egg Wrap

Makes 1 serving.

Eggs are a great way to work in the choline that is necessary to maximize your baby's brain growth and development.

2 eggs

2 tablespoons water

¼ cup red bell pepper or
cooked broccoli, asparagus, or
mushrooms, diced

1 7-inch whole-wheat tortilla

Salsa (optional)

In small bowl, beat together the eggs and water. Coat a 7-inch omelet pan with nonstick cooking spray and heat over medium-high heat. When the pan is hot, pour in the egg mixture. Tilt the pan to move the egg around until it covers the pan. When no visible liquid egg remains, sprinkle the top with the vegetables. Place the tortilla on a plate. Carefully slide the egg onto the tortilla. Roll it up and top with salsa, if desired.

Per Serving (without the salsa) Calories: 229 • Total fat: 11 grams • Saturated fat: 3 grams
Trans fat: n/a • Cholesterol: 423 milligrams • Sodium: 290 milligrams
Carbohydrate: 19 grams • Dietary fiber: 3 grams • Protein: 16 grams
Calcium: 60 milligrams • Iron: 3 milligrams

Salmon Burgers

Makes 2 servings.

It's easy to include in your diet the omega-3 fats and the high-quality protein that you and your baby require with these hearty burgers.

1 6½-ounce can salmon

2 tablespoons unseasoned bread crumbs

1 egg

½ tablespoon diced shallots

2 tablespoons diced red bell pepper

1 teaspoon dried dill

2 teaspoons canola oil

2 whole-grain sandwich buns

Lettuce (optional)

Sliced tomato (optional)

Place the salmon in a medium bowl and break it up with a fork. Add the bread crumbs, egg, shallots, bell pepper, and dill and combine well. Form the mixture into 2 burgers.

In a medium skillet, heat the oil over medium-high heat. Cook for about 4 minutes on each side. Serve on the sandwich buns with lettuce and tomato, if desired.

Per Serving (without the toppings) Calories: 503 • Total fat: 20 grams
Saturated fat: 4 grams • Trans fat: 1 gram • Cholesterol: 163 milligrams
Sodium: 625 milligrams • Carbohydrate: 41 grams • Dietary fiber: 6 grams
Protein: 35 grams • Calcium: 130 milligrams • Iron: 3 milligrams

---

Sloppy Turkey Joes

Makes 4 servings.

Here's another one that's so easy and so good for you, too. Use lean ground beef or ground pork for a change.

2 teaspoons canola oil

1 medium onion, peeled and chopped

8 ounces ground 100% lean turkey breast meat

1 8-ounce can diced tomatoes, undrained

3 tablespoons quick-cooking rolled oats

1 tablespoon Worcestershire sauce

4 whole-grain sandwich buns

In a large skillet, heat the oil. Add the onions and sauté until translucent. Add the turkey to the pan. Cook the meat and onions, constantly breaking the turkey into small pieces. Stir in the tomatoes, oats, and Worcestershire sauce. Bring the mixture to a boil, then reduce the heat. Simmer for 5 to 10 minutes, or until the mixture reaches the desired consistency. Serve on the sandwich buns.

Per Serving Calories: 462 • Total fat: 17 grams • Saturated fat: 5 grams • Trans fat: 1 gram • Cholesterol: 73 milligrams • Sodium: 598 milligrams • Carbohydrate: 43 grams Dietary fiber: 7 grams • Protein: 35 grams • Calcium: 130 milligrams • Iron: 5 milligrams

---

Portobello Mushroom Burgers

Makes 2 servings.

This is a simple alternative to beef burgers that won't leave you wanting for more.

2 large portobello mushroom caps

1 tablespoon olive or canola oil

Salt

Freshly ground black pepper

2 whole-grain sandwich buns

2 ounces reduced-fat, sliced cheddar cheese (optional)

Lettuce (optional)

Sliced tomato (optional)

Preheat the oven broiler or a grill. Brush the portobello caps with the oil. Sprinkle with salt and pepper. Broil or grill the mushrooms until tender, 5 to 10 minutes. Place the cooked mushrooms on a bun and top with cheese, lettuce, and tomato, if desired.

Per Serving (without the toppings) Calories: 337 • Total fat: 12 grams Saturated fat: 3 grams • Trans fat: 1 gram • Cholesterol: 6 milligrams Sodium: 573 milligrams • Carbohydrate: 39 grams • Dietary fiber: 7 grams Protein: 20 grams • Calcium: 210 milligrams • Iron: 4 milligrams

---

Roasted Red Pepper–Pesto Pita Pizza

Makes 2 servings.

This super-simple pie provides fiber and calcium, with a minimum of fuss.

½ cup part-skim ricotta cheese

2 tablespoons ready-made pesto sauce

2 large whole-wheat pita breads

¼ cup jarred roasted red peppers, drained

½ cup grated part-skim mozzarella cheese

1 teaspoon freshly ground black pepper (optional)

Preheat the oven to 375°F. In a small bowl, mix the ricotta cheese and pesto sauce. Spread half of the mixture on each pita bread. Top each bread with red peppers and mozzarella cheese. Season with black pepper, if desired. Bake for 5 minutes.

Per Serving Calories: 475 • Total fat: 25 grams • Saturated fat: 9 grams • Trans fat: n/a
Cholesterol: 34 milligrams • Sodium: 807 milligrams • Carbohydrate: 42 grams
Dietary fiber: 5 grams • Protein: 21 grams • Calcium: 380 milligrams
• Iron: 2 milligrams

FETA CHEESE AND SPINACH PIZZA
Makes 4 servings.

The prebaked crust in this recipe boosts your whole-grain intake while simplifying preparation.

2 teaspoons olive oil

8 ounces baby spinach, washed and dried

1 large prebaked whole-wheat pizza crust

⅓ cup grated Parmesan cheese

3 plum tomatoes, chopped

4 ounces feta cheese

Preheat the oven to 400°F. In a medium skillet, heat 1 teaspoon of the oil. Add the spinach and sauté until just wilted, about 2 minutes. Set aside.

Place the crust on an ungreased baking sheet. Sprinkle the crust with the remaining oil and the Parmesan cheese. Bake for 8 to 10 minutes.

Remove from the oven and top with the spinach, tomatoes, and feta cheese. Return to the oven and bake for 15 more minutes.

Per Serving Calories: 318 • Total fat: 10 grams • Saturated fat: 6 grams • Trans fat: n/a
Cholesterol: 32 milligrams • Sodium: 860 milligrams • Carbohydrate: 44 grams
Dietary fiber: 7 grams • Protein: 16 grams • Calcium: 300 milligrams
Iron: 4 milligrams

Quick Breads

FLUFFY PANCAKES

Makes 2 servings.

Start with a pancake mix and add yogurt to boost the calcium content.
Serve with applesauce instead of syrup to include a serving of fruit.

1 cup plain low-fat yogurt

1 egg

½ cup 1% low-fat milk

1 cup pancake mix

In a medium bowl, combine the yogurt, egg, and milk and mix well.

Add the pancake mix and stir until just moist. Lightly coat a griddle or a skillet with cooking spray and heat. Using a ¼ cup measure, pour the batter onto the hot griddle. Cook until the bubbles begin to burst, then flip and cook until golden brown.

Per serving (3 pancakes) Calories: 383 • Total fat: 8 grams
Saturated fat: 3 grams • Trans fat: n/a • Cholesterol: 126 milligrams
Sodium: 937 milligrams • Carbohydrate: 58 grams • Dietary fiber: 2 grams
Protein: 18 grams • Calcium: 470 milligrams • Iron: 3 milligrams

---

PUMPKIN PANCAKES

Makes 6 servings.

Pumpkin is rich in beta-carotene and other beneficial plant nutrients.
Leftover pancakes can be frozen and reheated for future use. Freeze
leftover canned pumpkin in a covered container. Use canned pumpkin
only, not pumpkin pie filling.

2 cups plain low-fat yogurt

¼ cup plus 1 tablespoon sugar

1⅔ cups flour

1 teaspoon baking soda

1 teaspoon cinnamon

½ teaspoon ground nutmeg

1 cup 1% low-fat milk

2 tablespoons trans fat–free
  tub margarine, melted

1 egg

½ cup canned pumpkin

In a small bowl, mix the yogurt with the ¼ cup of sugar. Set aside.

In a large bowl, combine the 1 tablespoon of sugar with the flour, baking soda, cinnamon, and nutmeg.

In a medium bowl, combine the milk, margarine, egg, pumpkin, and yogurt-sugar mixture, stirring well. Add the wet ingredients to the dry ingredients in the large bowl. Stir until it is moist and free of lumps.

Lightly coat a griddle or a skillet with nonstick cooking spray and heat to low to medium heat. Using a ¼ cup measure, pour the batter onto the hot griddle. Cook until the bubbles begin to burst, then flip and cook until golden brown.

Per Serving (3 pancakes) Calories: 282 • Total fat: 6 grams
Saturated fat: 3 grams • Trans fat: 0 • Cholesterol: 42 milligrams
Sodium: 198 milligrams • Carbohydrate: 45 grams • Dietary fiber: 3 grams
Protein: 12 grams • Calcium: 270 milligrams • Iron: 2 milligrams

---

CRANBERRY-NUT MUFFINS

Makes 12 servings.

These moist muffins substitute applesauce for some of the oil. They make great portable snacks.

1 cup unsweetened chunky applesauce	1 teaspoon ground cinnamon
⅓ cup canola oil	¼ teaspoon salt
2 cups all-purpose flour	½ cup dried cranberries
½ cup sugar	½ cup chopped walnuts
1 teaspoon baking soda	

Preheat the oven to 350°F. Line a muffin pan with paper liners or grease and flour the pan.

In a small bowl, combine the applesauce, oil, and egg. Set aside.

In a large bowl, combine the flour, sugar, baking soda, cinnamon, and salt. Add the wet ingredients to these dry ingredients and stir until just moistened. Gently fold in the cranberries and walnuts. Spoon the muffin mixture equally into the muffin cups.

Bake for 20 to 25 minutes, or until a toothpick inserted in the center comes out clean. Remove from the pan and cool on a rack.

Per Serving (1 muffin) Calories: 186 • Total fat: 10 grams • Saturated fat: 1 gram
Trans fat: 0 • Cholesterol: 18 milligrams • Sodium: 109 milligrams • Carbohydrate: 23 grams
Dietary fiber: 1 gram • Protein: 2 grams • Calcium: 10 milligrams • Iron: 1 milligram

---

Desserts and Snacks

YOGURT-BERRY PARFAIT

Makes 1 serving.

*This is simple, sweet, and very good for your bones
as well as your baby's.*

8 ounces plain low-fat yogurt

1 teaspoon sugar

½ cup fresh berries
(or frozen berries, thawed)

½ cup crunchy whole-grain
cereal, such as Wheat Chex

In a small bowl, mix the yogurt with the sugar. In a tall glass, place half
of the yogurt, half of the berries, and half of the cereal. Repeat.

Per Serving Calories: 313 • Total fat: 5 grams • Saturated fat: 3 grams • Trans fat: 0
Cholesterol: 15 milligrams • Sodium: 433 milligrams • Carbohydrate: 53 grams
Dietary fiber: 7 grams • Protein: 16 grams • Calcium: 530 milligrams • Iron: 9 milligrams

CHOCOLATE-RAISIN CLUSTERS

Makes 8 servings.

*If you're craving candy, have a couple of these fiber-filled dark chocolate
goodies. Use dried cranberries instead of raisins for a change of pace.*

6 ounces bittersweet chocolate chips

1 cup raisins

Melt the chocolate in the top of a double boiler, stirring constantly.
When it has melted, remove the top portion of the double boiler, set
asider, and turn off the burner. Add the raisins to the melted chocolate
and stir, completely coating the fruit. Using a teaspoon, drop the
chocolate-raisin mixture onto wax paper to form 16 clusters. Allow to
cool completely.

Per Serving (2 clusters) Calories: 170 • Total fat: 6 grams
Saturated fat: 4 grams • Trans fat: 0 • Cholesterol: 4 milligrams
Sodium: 2 milligrams • Carbohydrate: 30 grams • Dietary fiber: 2 grams
Protein: 2 grams • Calcium: 20 milligrams • Iron: 1 milligram

Popcorn Delight

Makes 1 serving.

Surprise! Popcorn is a whole grain. Work in a serving with this crunchy treat.

3 cups popped fat-free unsalted
  popcorn
1 tablespoon sliced almonds
2 tablespoons raisins or other
  dried fruit, such as cranberries,
  apricots, or dates

½ teaspoon ground cinnamon
1 teaspoon sugar

In a medium bowl, combine the ingredients and toss well.

Per Serving Calories: 230 • Total fat: 7 grams • Saturated fat: 1 gram • Trans fat: 0
Cholesterol: 0 Sodium: 274 milligrams • Carbohydrate: 39 grams
Dietary fiber: 6 grams • Protein: 6 grams • Calcium: 30 milligrams • Iron: 1 milligram

---

Caramel-Pear Sundae

Makes 1 serving.

Satisfy your sweet tooth with this healthy dessert.

2 canned pear halves
½ cup low-fat vanilla ice cream

2 tablespoons fat-free caramel sauce

Place the pears in a shallow dish. Top with the ice cream and caramel sauce.

Per Serving Calories: 328 • Total fat: 5 grams • Saturated fat: 3 grams • Trans fat: 0
Cholesterol: 26 milligrams • Sodium: 132 milligrams • Carbohydrate: 68
milligrams • Dietary fiber: 3 grams • Protein: 5 grams • Calcium: 160 milligrams • Iron: 0

No-Cook Nut Butter Crunchies

Makes 8 servings.

A cross between candy and cookie, these crunchy delights provide sweetness and heart-healthy fat. If you like, go nut-free with sunflower seed butter.

½ cup smooth almond, peanut, soy nut, or sunflower seed butter

½ cup honey

1 teaspoon vanilla extract

¾ cup powdered nonfat milk

⅔ cup crispy rice cereal

In a large bowl, blend the almond (or other) butter, honey, and vanilla. Add the powdered milk and cereal. Mix well and form into balls.

Per Serving (2 crunchies) Calories: 186 • Total fat: 8 grams • Saturated fat: 2 grams
Trans fat: 0 • Cholesterol: 2 milligrams • Sodium: 120 milligrams
Carbohydrate: 24 grams • Dietary fiber: 2 grams • Protein: 6 grams
Calcium: 40 milligrams • Iron: 1 milligram

BLUEBERRY CRISP

Makes 12 servings.

Blueberries are brimming with beneficial phytonutrients that protect you and your baby. Rolled oats and wheat germ add the goodness of grains.

Filling

5 cups fresh or frozen blueberries
(thaw before using)

Topping

½ cup packed brown sugar

¼ cup rolled oats, uncooked

¼ cup wheat germ

¼ teaspoon ground cinnamon

½ cup trans fat–free tub margarine

Preheat the oven to 375°F. Place the fruit in a 9 × 13 inch ungreased glass baking dish. In a medium bowl, combine the brown sugar, oats, wheat germ, and cinnamon. Cut in the margarine with a fork until the mixture resembles coarse crumbs. Sprinkle the brown sugar mixture over the top of the blueberries. Bake for 25 minutes, or until the fruit is tender. Cool before serving.

Per Serving Calories: 146 • Total fat: 7 grams • Saturated fat: 2 grams • Trans fat: 0
Cholesterol: 0 • Sodium: 64 milligrams • Carbohydrate: 21 grams • Dietary fiber: 2 grams
Protein: 2 grams • Calcium: 10 milligrams • Iron: 1 milligram

---

Resources

General

Academy of Neonatal Nursing
www.academyonline.org

American Academy of Family Physicians
www.aafp.org

American Academy of Nurse Practitioners
www.aanp.org

American Academy of Periodontology
www.perio.org

American College of Obstetricians and Gynecologists
www.acog.org

American Dietetic Association
www.eatright.org

American Gynecological Obstetrics Society
www.agosonline.org

American Physical Therapy Association
www.apta.org

Association of Women's Health, Obstetric, and Neonatal Nurses
www.awhonn.org

Canadian Women's Health Network
www.cwhn.ca

Centers for Disease Control and Prevention
www.cdc.gov/ncbddd/pregnancy_gateway/research.htm

Dietary Guidelines for Americans 2005
www.healthierus.gov/dietaryguidelines

Dietitians of Canada
www.dietitians.ca

March of Dimes
www.marchofdimes.com

National Association of Anorexia Nervosa and Associated Disorders
www.anad.org

National Birth Defects Prevention Network
www.nbdpn.org

National Domestic Violence Hotline
www.ndvh.org

National Eating Disorders Organization
www.nationaleatingdisorders.org

National Institute of Child Health and Development
www.nichd.nih.gov

Preeclampsia Foundation
www.preeclampsia.org/about.asp

Society for Maternal Fetal Medicine
www.smfm.org

Special Supplement Program for Women, Infants and Children (WIC)
www.fns.usda.gov/wic/Contacts/tollfreenumbers.htm

Women's Health Initiative and Office of Research on Women's Health
www.4women.gov/owh

Breastfeeding and Postpartum

Academy of Certified Childbirth Educators
www.acbe.com

American College of Nurse-Midwives
www.gotmom.org

Childbirth Education, International Childbirth Education Association
www.icea.org

International Lactation Consultant Association
www.ilca.org

La Leche League, International
www.llli.org

Postpartum Support International
www.postpartum.net

Sidelines National Support Network
www.sidelines.org

Food Safety

Centers for Disease Control and Prevention
www.cdc.gov/ncidod/dbmd/diseaseinfo/listeriosis_g.htm

Center for Food Safety and Nutrition, Food and Drug Administration
www.cfsan.fda.gov

Environmental Protection Agency, Safe Drinking Water Hotline
800-426-4791

Food and Drug Administration, Food Information Line
888-SAFE-FOOD

National Lead Information Center
www.epa.gov/lead

Natural Medicines Database
www.therapeuticresearch.com

U.S. Partnership for Food Safety Education
www.fightbac.org

Infertility

American Society of Reproductive Medicine
www.asrm.org

National Infertility Association
www.resolve.org

Midwives and Doulas

American College of Nurse-Midwives
www.midwife.org

Doulas of North America (DONA)
www.dona.org

Midwives Alliance of North America
www.mana.org

Multiple Births

Mothers of Supertwins (MOST)
www.mostonline.org

National Organization of Mothers of Twins Clubs
www.nomotc.org

Suggested Reading

The Busy Mom's Ultimate Fitness Guide by Cathy Moxley. InSight, 2006

The Complete Idiot's Guide to Feeding Your Baby and Toddler by Elizabeth M. Ward, MS, RD. Alpha Books, 2005

Gluten-Free Diet: A Comprehensive Resource Guide by Shelley Case, RD. Case Nutrition Consulting, 2006

Heading Home with Your Newborn: From Birth to Reality by Laura Jana, MD, and Jennifer Shu, MD. American Academy of Pediatrics, 2005

Lean Mommy by Lisa Druxman. Center Street, 2007

Managing Morning Sickness: A Survival Guide for Pregnant Women by Miriam Erick, MS, RD. Bull Publishing, 2004

New Mother's Guide to Breastfeeding by American Academy of Pediatrics. Bantam Books, 2002

Nursing Mother, Working Mother by Kathleen Huggins and Gale Pryor. Harvard Common Press, 2007

The Nursing Mother's Companion by Kathleen Huggins. Harvard Common Press, 2005

When You're Expecting Twins, Triplets or Quads: Proven Guidelines for a Healthy Multiple Pregnancy by Dr. Barbara Luke, MPH, RD, and Tamara Eberlein. HarperCollins, 2004

References

Introduction

Keller, G., et al. Nephron Number in Patients with Primary Hypertension. *New England Journal of Medicine* 348:101–108, 2003.

Position of the American Dietetic Association and Dietitians of Canada. Nutrition and Women's Health. *Journal of the American Dietetic Association* 104:984–1001, 2004.

U.S. Department of Health and Human Services. *The Health Consequences of Smoking: A Report of the Surgeon General—2004.* Atlanta, GA: Centers for Disease Control and Prevention, Office on Smoking and Health, 2004.

1. Prepregnancy: Starting from a Healthy Place

Allen, L. Multiple Micronutrients in Pregnancy and Lactation: An Overview. *American Journal of Clinical Nutrition* 81:1206S–1212S, 2005.

American Academy of Clinical Endocrinologists. Subclinical Hypothyroidism during Pregnancy: Position Statement from the American Association of Clinical Endocrinologists. www.aace.com/pub/pdf/guidelines/pregnancy.pdf.

American Academy of Pediatrics and the American College of Obstetricians and Gynecologists. *Guidelines for Perinatal Care*, 5th ed. Elk Grove Village, IL: Authors, 2002.

American Academy of Periodontology. Baby Steps to a Healthy Pregnancy and On-Time Delivery. www.perio.org/consumer/pregnancy.htm.

American Cancer Society. Neuroblastoma. www.cancer.org.

American College of Obstetricians and Gynecologists. Good Health before Pregnancy. www.acog.org/publications/patient_education/bpo56.cfm.

―――. Smoking Cessation during Pregnancy. *Obstetrics and Gynecology* 106:883–888, 2005.

American Diabetes Association. Standards of Medical Care in Diabetes—2007. *Diabetes Care* 30:S4-S41, 2007.

―――. www.diabetes.org.

American Dietetic Association. Position of the American Dietetic Association: Nutrition and Lifestyle for a Healthy Pregnancy Outcome. *Journal of the American Dietetic Association* 108:553–561, 2008.

American Pregnancy Association. Drinking Herbal Teas during Pregnancy. www.americanpregnancy.org/pregnancyhealth/herbaltea.html.

American Thyroid Association. Hypothryroidism. www.thyroid.org/patients/brochures/Hypothyroidism%20_web_booklet.pdf.

Bailey, L., and Berry, R. Folic Acid Supplementation and the Occurrence of Congenital Heart Defects, Orofacial Clefts, Multiple Births, and Miscarriage. *American Journal of Clinical Nutrition* 81:1213S–1217S, 2005.

Bergholt, T., et al. Maternal Body Mass Index in the First Trimester and Risk of Cesarean Delivery in Nulliparous Women in Spontaneous Labor. *American Journal of Obstetrics & Gynecology* 96:163e1–163e5, 2007.

Berry, R., et al. Prevention of Neural Tube Defects with Folic Acid in China. *New England Journal of Medicine* 341:1485–1490, 1999.

Carmichael, S., et al. Physical Activity and Risk of Neural Tube Defects. *Maternal and Child Health Journal* 6:151–157, 2002.

Centers for Disease Control and Prevention. Folic Acid: Frequently Asked Questions. www.cdc.gov/ncbddd/folicacid/faqs.htm.

―――. National Center on Birth Defects and Developmental Disabilities. www.cdc.gov/ncbddd.

————. Recommendations to Improve Preconception Health and Health Care—United States. *Morbidity and Mortality Weekly Report* 55, April 21, 2006.

————. Vaccinations. wwwn.cdc.gov/travel/contentVaccinations.aspx.

Day, N., et al. Prenatal Alcohol Exposure Predicts Continued Deficits in Offspring Size at 14 Years of Age. *Alcoholism: Clinical and Experimental Research* 26:1584–1591, 2002.

Dempsey, J. Prospective Study of Gestational Diabetes Mellitus Risk in Relationship to Maternal Recreational Physical Activity Before and During Pregnancy. *American Journal of Epidemiology* 159:663–670, 2004.

Dietary Guidelines for Americans 2005. Adequate Nutrients within Calorie Needs. www.health.gov/dietaryguidelines/dga2005/document/html/chapter2.htm.

Fasano, A. et al. Prevalence of Celiac Disease in At-Risk and Not-At-Risk Groups in the United States: A Large Multicenter Study. *Archives of Internal Medicine* 163:286–292, 2003.

Gensink Law, D. Obesity and Time to Pregnancy. *Human Reproduction.* 22:414–420, 2007.

Goh, Y. I., et al. Prenatal Multivitamin Supplementation and Rates of Congenital Anomalies: A Meta-Analysis. *Journal of Obstetrics and Gynaecology of Canada* 28:680–689, 2006.

Haddow, J., et al. Maternal Thyroid Deficiency during Pregnancy and Subsequent Neuropsychological Development of the Child. *New England Journal of Medicine* 341:549–555, 1999.

Hooiveld, M., et al. Adverse Reproductive Outcomes among Male Painters with Occupational Exposure to Organic Solvents. *Occupational and Environmental Medicine* 63:538–544, 2006.

Jensen, T., et al. Body Mass Index in Relation to Semen Quality and Reproductive Hormones among 1,558 Danish Men. *Fertility and Sterility* 82:863–870, 2004.

Ji, B., et al. Paternal Cigarette Smoking and the Risk of Childhood Cancer among Offspring of Nonsmoking Mothers. *Journal of the National Cancer Institute* 89:238–244, 1997.

Kesmodel, U., et al. Moderate Alcohol Intake during Pregnancy and the Risk of Stillbirth and Death in the First Year of Life. *American Journal of Epidemiology* 155:305–312, 2002.

Li, D. K., et al. Exposure to Non-Steroidal Anti-Inflammatory Drugs during Pregnancy and Risk of Miscarriage: Population Based Cohort Study. *British Medical Journal* 327:386, 2003.

Lu, M. Recommendations for Preconception Care. *American Family Physician* 76:397–400, 2007.

March of Dimes. Caffeine in Pregnancy. www.marchofdimes.com/professionals/14332_1148.asp.

———. Drinking Alcohol during Pregnancy. www.marchofdimes.com/professionals/14332_1170.asp.

———.Smoking during Pregnancy. www.marchofdimes.com/printable Articles/14332_1171.asp.

———. Vaccinations during Pregnancy. www.marchofdimes.com/print ableArticles/159_16189.asp.

Ray, J., et al. Greater Maternal Weight and the Ongoing Risk of Neural Tube Defects after Folic Acid Flour Fortification. *Obstetrics and Gynecology* 105:261–265, 2005.

Salihu, H., et al. Extreme Obesity and Risk of Stillbirth among Black and White Gravidas. *Obstetrics & Gynecology* 110:552–557, 2007.

Scholl, T. Iron Status during Pregnancy: Setting the Stage for Mother and Infant. *American Journal of Clinical Nutrition* 81:1218S–1222S, 2005.

Sokol, R., et al. Fetal Alcohol Spectrum Disorder. *Journal of the American Medical Association* 290:2996–2999, 2003.

Sood, B., et al. Prenatal Alcohol Exposure and Childhood Behavior at Age 6 to 7. *Pediatrics* 108:e34, 2001.

Streissguth, A. P., et al. Risk Factors for Adverse Life Outcomes in Fetal Alcohol Syndrome and Fetal Alcohol Effects. *Journal of Developmental and Behavioral Pediatrics* 25:228–238, 2004.

Vahratian, A., et al. Multivitamin Use and the Risk of Preterm Birth. *American Journal of Epidemiology* 160:886–892, 2004.

Vergnes, J. N., and Sixou, M. Preterm Low Birth Weight and Maternal Periodontal Status: A Meta-Analysis. *American Journal of Obstetrics & Gynecology* 196:135e1–135e7, 2007.

Waller, D., et al. Prepregnancy Obesity as a Risk Factor for Structural Birth Defects, *Archives of Pediatriac and Adolescent Medicine* 161:745–750, 2007.

Wallock, L., et al. Low Seminal Plasma Folate Concentrations Are Associated with Low Sperm Density and Count in Male Smokers and Nonsmokers. *Fertility and Sterility* 75:252–259, 2001.

Wang, J. Body Mass and Probability of Pregnancy during Assisted Reproduction Treatment: Retrospective Study. *British Medical Journal* 321:1320–1321, 2000.

Wilcox, A. J., et al. Folic Acid Supplements and the Risk of Facial Clefts: A National Population-Based Case-Control Study. *British Medical Journal* 334:464, 2007.

2. Great Expectations: How Eating the Right Food Is Good for You and Your Baby

American Academy of Pediatrics. *Pediatric Nutrition Handbook*, 5th ed. Elk Grove Village, IL: Authors, 2004.

———. Committee on Drugs. Policy Statement: The Transfer of Drugs and Other Chemicals into Human Milk. *Pediatrics,* 108:776–789, 2001.

American Academy of Pediatrics and American College of Obstetricians and Gynecologists. *Guidelines for Perinatal Care,* 5th ed. Elk Grove Village, IL: Authors, 2002.

American College of Obstetricians and Gynecologists. *Your Pregnancy and Birth,* 4th ed. Washington, DC: Authors, 2005.

American Dietetic Association. Position of the American Dietetic Association: Nutrition and Lifestyle for a Healthy Pregnancy Outcome. *Journal of the American Dietetic Association* 108:553–561, 2008.

Batres-Marquez, S. P., et al. Choline in the Diets of the U.S. Population: NHANES 2003–2004. Abstract presented at the Conference of Experimental Biology, 2007.

Berry, R. J., et al. Prevention of Neural Tube Defects with Folic Acid in China. *New England Journal of Medicine* 341:1485–1490, 1999.

Bodnar, L., et al. High Prevalence of Vitamin D Insufficiency in Black and White Pregnant Women Residing in the Northern United States and Their Neonates. *Journal of Nutrition* 137:447–452, 2007.

———. Maternal Vitamin D Deficiency Increases the Risk of Preeclampsia. *Journal of Clinical Endocrinology & Metabolism* 92: 3517–3522, 2007.

Camargo, C., et al. Maternal Intake of Vitamin D during Pregnancy and Risk of Recurrent Wheeze in Children at 3 Years of Age. *American Journal of Clinical Nutrition* 85:788–795, 2007.

Cannell, J., et al. Epidemic Influenza and Vitamin D. *Epidemiology and Infection* 134:1129–1140, 2006.

Centers for Disease Control and Prevention. Folic Acid. cdc.gov/ncbddd/folicacid.

Cnattingus, S., et al. Caffeine Intake and the Risk of First-Trimester Spontaneous Abortion. *New England Journal of Medicine* 25:1839–1845, 2000.

Dietary Guidelines for Americans 2005. Sodium and Potassium. www.health.gov/dietaryguidelines/dga2005/document/html/chapter8.htm.

Feskanich, D., et al. Vitamin A Intake and Hip Fractures among Postmenopausal Women. *Journal of the American Medical Association* 287:47–54, 2002.

Garland, C., et al. Role of Ultraviolet B Irradiance and Vitamin D in Prevention of Ovarian Cancer. *American Journal of Preventive Medicine* 31:512–514, 2006.

Hernandez-Diaz, S., et al. Folic Acid Antagonists during Pregnancy and the Risk of Birth Defects. *New England Journal of Medicine* 343:1608–1614, 2000.

Innis, S., et al. Essential Omega-3 Fatty Acids in Pregnant Women and Early Visual Acuity Maturation in Term Infants. *American Journal of Clinical Nutrition* 87:548–557, 2008.

John, E., et al. Vitamin D and Breast Cancer Risk: The NHANES I Epidemiologic Follow-Up Study, 1971–1975 to 1992. National Health and Examination Survey. *Cancer Epidemiology, Biomarkers & Prevention* 8:399–406, 1999.

Johnson, L., et al. Reproductive Defects Are Corrected in Vitamin D–Deficient Female Rats Fed a High Calcium, Phosphorus and Lactose Diet. *Journal of Nutrition* 132:2270–2273, 2002.

Klebanoff, M., et al. Maternal Serum Paraxanthine, a Caffeine Metabolite, and the Risk of Spontaneous Abortion. *New England Journal of Medicine* 341:1639–1644, 1999.

Koletzko, B., et al. Dietary Fat Intakes for Pregnant and Lactating Women. *British Journal of Nutrition* 98:873–877, 2007.

Makrides, J., et al. Fatty Acid Composition of Brain, Retina, and Erythrocytes in Breast- and Formula-Fed Infants. *American Journal of Clinical Nutrition* 60:189–194, 1994.

March of Dimes. Caffeine in Pregnancy. www.marchofdimes.com/professionals/14332_1148.asp.

———. Folic Acid. www.marchofdimes.com/professionals/690_1399.asp.

Munger, K., et al. Serum 25-Hydroxyvitamin D Levels and Risk of Multiple Sclerosis. *Journal of the American Medical Association* 296:2832–2838, 2006.

National Academies of Science. Institute of Medicine. Food and Nutrition Board. *Dietary Reference Intakes for Calcium, Phosphorus, Magnesium, Vitamin D, and Fluoride.* Washington, DC: National Academies Press, 1997.

———. *Dietary Reference Intakes for Energy, Carbohydrate, Fiber, Fat, Fatty Acids, Cholesterol, Protein, and Amino Acids.* Washington, DC: National Academies Press, 2002.

———. *Dietary Reference Intakes for Thiamin, Riboflavin, Niacin, Vitamin B_6, Folate, Vitamin B_{12}, Pantothenic Acid, Biotin, and Choline.* Washington, DC: National Academies Press, 2000.

———. *Dietary Reference Intakes for Vitamin A, Vitamin K, Arsenic, Boron, Chromium, Copper, Iodine, Iron, Manganese, Molybdenum, Nickel, Silicon, Vanadium, and Zinc.* Washington, DC: National Academies Press, 2001.

———. *Dietary Reference Intakes for Vitamin C, Vitamin E, Selenium, and Carotenoids.* Washington, DC: National Academies Press, 2000.

———. *Dietary Reference Intakes for Water, Potassium, Sodium, Chloride, and Sulfate.* Washington, DC: National Academies Press, 2004.

National Institutes of Health. National Library of Medicine. Medline Plus. Iodine in Diet. www.nlm.nih.gov/medlineplus/ency/article/002421.htm.

———. Vitamin K. www.nlm.nih.gov/medlineplus/druginfo/natural/patient- vitamink.html.

———. Office of Dietary Supplements. Dietary Supplement Fact Sheet: Calcium. www.dietary-supplements.info.nih.gov/factsheets/calcium.asp.

———. Dietary Supplement Fact Sheet: Magnesium. www.dietary-supplements.info.nih.gov/factsheets/magnesium.asp.

————. Dietary Supplement Fact Sheet: Vitamin A and Carotenoids. www.ods.od.nih.gov/factsheets/vitamina.asp.

————. Dietary Supplement Fact Sheet: Vitamin E. www.ods.od.nih .gov/factsheets/vitamine.asp.

Nelen, W., et al. Homocysteine and Folate Levels as Risk Factors for Recurrent Early Pregnancy Loss. *Obstetrics & Gynecology* 95:519–524, 2000.

Rothman, K., et al. Teratogenicity of High Vitamin A Intake. *New England Journal of Medicine* 33:1369–1373, 1995.

Savitz, D., et al. Caffeine and Miscarriage Risk. *Epidemiology* 19:55–62, 2008.

Shaw, G., et al. Periconceptional Dietary Intake of Choline and Betaine and Neural Tube Defects in Offspring. *American Journal of Epidemiology* 160:102–109, 2004.

Siega-Riz, A., et al. Second Trimester Folate Status and Preterm Birth. *American Journal of Obstetrics and Gynecology* 191:1851–1857, 2004.

Simopoulos, A., et al. Workshop on the Essentiality of and Recommended Dietary Intakes for Omega-6 and Omega-3 Fatty Acids. *Journal of the American College of Nutrition* 18:487–489, 1999.

U.S. Department of Agriculture. Nutrient Data Laboratory. www.ars .usda.gov/main/site_main.htm?modecode=12354500.

U.S. Department of Health and Human Services. Advance Data from Vital and Health Statistics. Dietary Intake of Selected Vitamins for the United States Population: 1999–2000. Centers for Disease Control and Prevention. National Center for Health Statistics 339, 2004.

Weng, X., et al. Maternal Caffeine Consumption during Pregnancy and the Risk of Miscarriage: A Prospective Cohort Study. *American Journal of Obstetrics and Gynecology* 198:279.e1–279.e8, 2008.

Wisborg, K., et al. Maternal Consumption of Coffee during Pregnancy and Stillbirth and Infant Death in the First Year of Life: Prospective Study. *British Medical Journal* 326:420–423, 2003.

Zeisel, S. Nutritional Importance of Choline for Brain Development. *Journal of the American College of Nutrition* 23:621S-626S, 2004.

3. MyPyramind Plans: What to Eat Before, During, and After Pregnancy

Dietary Guidelines for Americans 2005. Background and Purpose of the Dietary Guidelines for Americans. www.health.gov/dietary guidelines.

National Academies of Science. Institute of Medicine. Food and Nutrition Board. *Dietary Reference Intakes for Energy, Carbohydrate, Fiber, Fat, Fatty Acids, Cholesterol, Protein, and Amino Acids.* Washington, DC: National Academies Press, 2002.

U. S. Department of Agriculture. MyPyramid.gov.

4. Pregnancy: Expect the Best

American Academy of Pediatrics. Breastfeeding and the Use of Human Milk: Policy Statement. *Pediatrics* 115:496–506, 2005.

American Academy of Pediatrics and American College of Obstetricians and Gynecologists. *Guidelines for Perinatal Care*, 5th ed.. Elk Grove Village, IL: Authors, 2002.

American College of Obstetricians and Gynecologists. *Repeated Miscarriage*. ACOG Education Pamphlet AP100. Washington, DC: Authors, 2000.

———. *Your Pregnancy and Birth*, 4th ed. Washington, DC: Authors, 2005.

American Dietetic Association. *ADA Nutrition Care Manual*. www .nutritioncaremanual.org.

———. Position of the American Dietetic Association: Nutrition and Lifestyle for a Healthy Pregnancy Outcome. *Journal of the American Dietetic Association* 108:553–561, 2008.

———. Position of the American Dietetic Association: Promoting and Supporting Breastfeeding. *Journal of the American Dietetic Association* 105:810–818, 2005.

Artal, R., et al. A Lifestyle Intervention of Weight-Gain Restriction: Diet and Exercise in Obese Women with Gestational Diabetes. *Applied Physiology in Nutrition and Metabolism* 32:596–601, 2007.

Artal, R., and O'Toole, M. Guidelines of the American College of Obstetricians and Gynecologists for Exercise during Pregnancy and the Postpartum Period. *British Journal of Sports Medicine* 37:6–12, 2003.

Bayol S., et al. A Maternal "Junk Food" Diet in Pregnancy and Lactation Promotes an Exacerbated Taste for "Junk Food" and a Greater Propensity for Obesity in Rat Offspring. *British Journal of Nutrition*, 98:843-851, 2007.

Clapp, J., et al. Beginning Regular Exercise in Early Pregnancy: Effect on Fetoplacental Growth. *American Journal of Obstetrics & Gynecology* 183:1484–1488, 2000.

de La Rochebrochard, E., and Thonneau, P. Paternal Age and Maternal Age Are Risk Factors for Miscarriage: Results of a Multicentre European Study. *Human Reproduction* 17:1649–1656, 2002.

Greer, F., et al. Effects of Early Nutritional Interventions on the Development of Atopic Disease in Infants and Children: The Role of Maternal Dietary Restriction, Breastfeeding, Timing of Introduction of Complementary Foods, and Hydrolyzed Formulas. *Pediatrics*, 1:183–191, 2008.

Hogge, W. A. The Clinical Use of Karyotyping Spontaneous Abortions. *American Journal of Obstetrics and Gynecology* 189:397–402, 2003.

Kiel, D., et al. Gestational Weight Gain and Pregnancy Outcomes in Obese Women: How Much Is Enough? *Obstetrics and Gynecology* 110:752–758, 2007.

Klein, L. Nutritional Recommendations for Multiple Pregnancies. *Journal of the American Dietetic Association* 105:1050–1052, 2005.

Koletzko, B., et al. Dietary Fat Intakes for Pregnant and Lactating Women. *British Journal of Nutrition* 98:873–877, 2007.

Kris-Etheron, P., and Innis, S. Position of the American Dietetic Association and Dietitians of Canada: Dietary Fatty Acids. *Journal of the American Dietetic Association* 107:1599–1611, 2007.

March of Dimes. Miscarriage. www.marchofdimes.com/professionals/ 14332_1192.asp.

National Academies of Science. Institute of Medicine. *Nutrition during Pregnancy*. Washington, DC: National Academies Press, 1990.

———. Institute of Medicine. Food and Nutrition Board. *Dietary Reference Intakes for Energy, Carbohydrate, Fiber, Fat, Fatty Acids, Cholesterol, Protein, and Amino Acids*. Washington, DC: National Academies Press, 2002.

———. Institute of Medicine. Food and Nutrition Board. *Dietary Reference Intakes for Vitamin A, Vitamin K, Arsenic, Boron, Chromium, Copper,*

Iodine, Iron, Manganese, Molybdenum, Nickel, Silicon, Vanadium, and Zinc. Washington, DC: National Academies Press, 2001.

———. National Research Council and Institute of Medicine. *Influence of Pregnancy Weight on Maternal and Child Health: Workshop Report.* Washington, DC: National Academies Press, 2007.

National Institutes of Health. National Library of Medicine. Medline Plus. Fetal Development. www.nlm.nih.gov/medlineplus/ency/article/002398.htm.

———. Fetus (12 Weeks Old). www.nlm.nih.gov/medlineplus/ency/imagepages/9572.htm.

———. Miscarriage. www.nlm.nih.gov.sapl.sat.lib.tx.us/medlineplus/ency/article/001488.htm.

Scholl, T. Iron Status during Pregnancy: Setting the Stage for Mother and Infant. *American Journal of Clinical Nutrition* 81:1218S–1222S, 2005.

Simopoulos, A., et al. Workshop on the Essentiality of and Recommended Dietary Intakes for Omega-6 and Omega-3 Fatty Acids. *Journal of the American College of Nutrition* 18:487–489, 1999.

5. The Fourth Trimester: After the Baby Arrives

Ainsworth, B., et al. Compendium of Physical Activities: An Update of Activity Codes and MET Intensities. *Medicine & Science in Sports and Exercise* 32:S498-504, 2000.

American Academy of Pediatrics. *Pediatric Nutrition Handbook,* 5th ed. Elk Grove Village, IL: Authors, 2004.

American College of Sports Medicine Roundtable Consensus Statement. Impact of Physical Activity during Pregnancy and Postpartum on Chronic Disease Risk. *Medicine & Science in Sports & Exercise* 38:989–1006, 2006.

Artal, R., and O'Toole, M. Guidelines of the American College of Obstetricians and Gynecologists for Exercise during Pregnancy and the Postpartum Period. *British Journal of Sports Medicine* 37:6–12, 2003.

Barr, R. Colic and Crying Syndrome in Infants. *Pediatrics* 102:1282–1286, 1998.

Chavez, G. Mental Health Policy Panel CCFC, April 18, 2002. California Department of Health Services. www.ccfc.ca.gov/PDF/SRI/DrChavez.pdf.

Garrison M., and Christakis, D. A Systematic Review of Treatments for Infant Colic. *Pediatrics* 106(1):184–190, 2000.

Hinton, P., and Olson, C. Postpartum Exercise and Food Intake: The Importance of Behavior-Specific Self-Efficacy. *Journal of the American Dietetic Association* 101:1430–1437, 2001.

Koletzko, B., et al. Dietary Fat Intakes for Pregnant and Lactating Women. *British Journal of Nutrition* 98:873–877, 2007.

National Institutes of Health. National Library of Medicine. Medline Plus. Colic and Crying. www.nlm.nih.gov/medlineplus/ency/article/000978.htm.

Postpartum Support International. Supporting Postpartum Families. www.postpartum.net.

Simopoulos, A., et al. Workshop on the Essentiality of and Recommended Dietary Intakes for Omega-6 and Omega-3 Fatty Acids. *Journal of the American College of Nutrition* 18:487–489, 1999.

Wagner, C., and Greer, F. Prevention of Rickets and Vitamin D Deficiency in Infants, Children, and Adolescents. *Pediatrics* 122:1142–1152, 2008.

Williamson, D., et al. The 10-year Incidence of Overweight and Major Weight Gain in U.S. Adults. *Archives of Internal Medicine* 150:665–672, 1990.

6. Food Safety: Before, During, and After Pregnancy

Agency for Toxic Substances and Disease Registry (ATSDR). Polychlorinated Biphenlys. www.atsdr.cdc.gov/substances/PCBs/index.html.

Bakardjiev A. I., Theriot J. A., and Portnoy D. A. *Listeria monocytogenes* Traffics from Maternal Organs to the Placenta and Back. *PLoS Pathogens* 2(6): 623–631, 2006.

Centers for Disease Control and Prevention. *CDC's Third National Report on Human Exposure to Environmental Chemicals: Spotlight on Dioxins, Furans, and Dioxin-Like Polychlorinated Biphenyls.* www.cdc.gov/exposurereport/pdf/factsheet_dioxinsfurans.pdf.

———. *Escherichia coli* O157:H7. www.cdc.gov/ncidod/dbmd/diseaseinfo/escherichiacoli_g.htm.

———. Lead Exposure among Females of Childbearing Age—United States, 2004. *Morbidity and Mortality Weekly* 56:397–400, 2007. www.cdc.gov/mmwr/preview/mmwrhtml/mm5616a4.htm.

————. Preventing Congenital Toxoplasmosis. *Morbidity and Mortality Weekly Report* 498, March 21, 2000.

————. Salmonellosis. www.cdc.gov/ncidod/dbmd/diseaseinfo/salmonel losis_g.htm.

Environmental Protection Agency. Is There Lead in My Drinking Water? www.epa.gov/safewater/lead/leadfactsheet.html.

Food and Drug Administration. Center for Food Safety and Applied Nutrition. Before You're Pregnant. www.cfsan.fda.gov/~pregnant/bef methy.html.

Hibbeln, J., et al. Maternal Seafood Consumption in Pregnancy and Neurodevelopmental Outcomes in Childhood (ALSPAC Study): An Observational Cohort Study. *The Lancet* 369:578–585, 2007.

March of Dimes. Environmental Risks and Pregnancy. www.marchofdimes/com/printableArticles/14332_9146.asp.

Organization of Teratology Information Specialists. Lead and Pregnancy. www.otispregnancy.org/pdf/lead.pdf.

7. Infertility, Other Common Concerns, and Special Situations

American College of Gastroenterology. Heartburn and GERD FAQ. www.acg.gi.org/patients/gerd/faqansw.asp.

American Diabetes Association. Gestational Diabetes. www.diabetes .org/gestational-diabetes.jsp.

American Dietetic Association. Position of the American Dietetic Association: Nutrition and Lifestyle for a Healthy Pregnancy Outcome. *Journal of the American Dietetic Association* 108:553–561, 2008.

American Society for Reproductive Medicine. Infertility. www.asrm.org/Patients/faqs.html.

————. Nutrition and Reproductive Health. www.asrm.org/Media/Press/nutrition.html.

Bodnar, L., et al. Periconceptual Multivitamin Use Reduces the Risk of Preeclampsia. *American Journal of Epidemiology* 164:470–477, 2006.

Burkman, L. J. Marijuana Impacts Sperm Function Both In Vivo and In Vitro: Semen Analyses from Men Smoking Marijuana. Conference of the American Society of Reproductive Medicine, San Antonio, TX, October 11–15, 2003.

Centers for Disease Control and Prevention. Births: Preliminary Data for 2006. *National Vital Statistics Reports* 56(7), December 5, 2007.

Chavarro, J., et al. Dietary Fatty Acid Intakes and the Risk of Ovulatory Infertility. *American Journal of Clinical Nutrition* 85:231–237, 2007.

Correa-Pérez, J. Smoking and Sperm Viability—a Never-Ending Story. *Fertility and Sterility* 79:1469, 2003.

Getahun, D., et al. Primary Preeclampsia in the Second Pregnancy: Effects of Changes in Prepregnancy Body Mass Index between Pregnancies. *Obstetrics and Gynecology* 110:1319–1325, 2007.

Heinrichs, L. Linking Olfaction with Nausea and Vomiting of Pregnancy, Recurrent Abortion, Hyperemesis Gravidarum, and Migraine Headache. *American Journal of Obstetrics & Gynecology* 186: S215-S219, 2002.

Hofmeyr, G., et al. Dietary Calcium Supplementation for Prevention of Pre-eclampsia and Related Problems: A Systematic Review and Commentary. *British Journal of Obstetrics and Gynaecology* 8:933–943, 2007.

March of Dimes. Multiples: Twins, Triplets, and Beyond. www.march ofdimes/printableArticles/14332_4545.asp.

National Institute of Diabetes and Digestive and Kidney Disorders. Constipation. www.digestive.niddk.nih.gov/ddiseases/pubs/constipation.

National Institutes Consensus Development Conference on Celiac Disease, 2004. Consensus.nih.gov/2004/2004CeliacDisease118html.htm.

National Institutes of Health. National Library of Medicine. Medline Plus. Morning Sickness. www.nlm.nih.gov/medlineplus/ency/article/003119.htm.

Nguyen, R. Men's Body Mass Index and Infertility. *Human Reproduction*. 22:2488–2493, 2007.

O'Brien, K., et al. Calcium Absorption Is Significantly Higher in Adolescents during Pregnancy Than in the Early Postpartum Period. *American Journal of Clinical Nutrition* 78:1188–1193, 2003.

Quinlan, J. Nausea and Vomiting of Pregnancy. *American Family Physician* 68:121–128, 2003.

Saleh, R., et al. Effect of Cigarette Smoking on Levels of Seminal Oxidative Stress in Infertile Men: A Prospective Study. *Fertility and Sterility* 78:491–499, 2002.

Sartorelli, E., et al. Effect of Paternal Age on Human Sperm Chromosomes. *Fertility and Sterility* 76:1119–1123, 2001.

Scholl, T. Oxidative Stress, Diet, and the Etiology of Preeclampsia *American Journal of Clinical Nutrition* 81:1390–1396, 2005.

Sheynkin, Y., et al. Increase in Scrotal Temperature in Laptop Computer Users. *Human Reproduction* 18:374–383, 2003.

U.S. Department of Health and Human Services. Polycystic Ovary Syndrome. www.4woman.gov/faq/pcos.htm.

Wen, S., et al. Folic Acid Supplementation in Early Second Trimester and the Risk of Preeclampsia. *American Journal of Obstetrics & Gynecology* 198:45.e1–45.e7, 2008.

Wong, W., et al. Effects of Folic Acid and Zinc Sulfate on Male Factor Subfertility: A Double-Blind, Randomized, Placebo-Controlled Trial. *Fertility and Sterility* 77:491–498, 2002.

———. Male Factor Subfertility: Possible Causes and the Impact of Nutritional Factors. *Fertility and Sterility* 73:435–442, 2000.

Wright, V., et al. Assisted Reproductive Technology Surveillance—2003. *Morbidity and Mortality Weekly Report* 55, May 26, 2006.

Yazigi, R., et al. Demonstration of Specific Binding of Cocaine to Human Spermatozoa. *Journal of the American Medical Association* 266:1956–1959, 1991.

Index